Paula Smith.

Special Tests a

SPECIAL TESTS
AND
THEIR MEANINGS

D. M. D. Evans

MD, FRCP, FRCPATH
Consultant Pathologist to the
South Glamorgan Health Authority (Teaching)
based at Llandough Hospital

Twelfth Edition

FABER AND FABER
London & Boston

First published in 1939
by Faber and Faber Limited
3 Queen Square London WC1N 3AU
New editions 1945, 1948, 1955, 1960, 1964, 1969,
1971, 1973, 1976, 1978
Twelfth edition 1981
Printed in Great Britain by
Fakenham Press Limited, Fakenham, Norfolk

British Library Cataloguing in Publication Data

Evans, D. M. D
Special tests and their meanings.—
12th ed.
1. Diagnosis
2. Medicine, Clinical—Laboratory manuals
I. Title
616.07′5   RB37

ISBN 0–571–18034–5

Preface to the Twelfth Edition

Many new and sensitive methods of biological investigation have been made available to hospital patients with the development of the Supraregional Assay Service (SAS). This greatly extends the range of the medical biochemistry departments. Some of the more complex (and expensive) investigations are in the field of hormone assay for endocrine disorders. The assays of proteins, blood lead and tissue enzymes are also available through this service. The range of these investigations has necessitated expansion of this book in order to outline the scope and requirements of this new generation of special tests.

January 1981   D. M. D. Evans

Acknowledgements

In preparing this twelfth edition I am indebted to Dr M. D. Crane, radiologist; Mr K. Tomlinson, Mr B. P. Spragg and Mr P. Henry, biochemists; Dr R. P. M. Marks, medical biochemist; Dr A. H. Quoraishi, medical microbiologist; Dr A. Evans, virologist; Mrs M. C. Makepeace, pharmacist and Drs C. D. and R. A. Evans, hospital doctors, for their helpful suggestions.

David Evans

Abbreviations Used

SAS = Supraregional Assay Service

h = hour(s)

m = minute(s)

sec = second(s)

< = less than

> = greater than

IV = intravenous

iu = International Unit

mU = milliUnit (a thousandth of a Unit)

mol = mole (for molecular substances this is the molecular weight in grammes)

mmol = millimole (a thousandth of a mole)

μmol = micromole (a millionth of a mole)

nmol = nanomole (a thousandth of a millionth of a mole)

pmol = picomole (a millionth of a millionth of a mole)

dl = decilitre (one tenth of a litre)

  = litre $\times 10^{-1}$, i.e. $\dfrac{\text{litre}}{10}$

ml = millilitre (a thousandth of a litre). For practical purposes this is equal to a cubic centimetre (cm^3)

fl = femtolitre (a thousandth of a millionth of a millionth of a litre)

  = litre $\times 10^{-15}$, i.e. $\dfrac{\text{litre}}{1\,000\,000\,000\,000\,000}$

kg = kilogramme (a thousand grammes) = $g \times 10^3$

g = gramme

mg = a milligramme (a thousandth of a gramme)

  = $g \times 10^{-3}$, i.e. $\dfrac{g}{1\,000}$

Abbreviations Used

μg = microgramme (a millionth of a gramme)

= g×10^{-6}, i.e. $\dfrac{g}{1\,000\,000}$

ng = nanogramme (a thousandth of a millionth of a gramme)

= g×10^{-9}, i.e. $\dfrac{g}{1\,000\,000\,000}$

pg = picogramme (a millionth of a millionth of a gramme)

= g×10^{-12}, i.e. $\dfrac{g}{1\,000\,000\,000\,000}$

m = metre

cm = centimetre (a hundredth of a metre)

= m×10^{-2}, i.e. $\dfrac{m}{100}$

mm = millimetre (a thousandth of a metre)

= m×10^{-3}, i.e. $\dfrac{m}{1\,000}$

mm^3 = cubic millimetre

μm = micrometre (a millionth of a metre)

= m×10^{-6}, i.e. $\dfrac{m}{1\,000\,000}$

nm = nanometre (a thousandth of a millionth of a metre)

= m×10^{-9}, i.e. $\dfrac{m}{1\,000\,000\,000}$. Nanometre is the unit of measurement of light wavelength

osmol/kg

= osmotic pressure exerted by 1 mole of substance in 1 kilogramme of solvent

mosm/kg

= osmotic pressure exerted by 1 millimole of a substance in 1 kilogramme

Unit being replaced

mEq = milli-equivalent (a thousandth of the equivalent weight in grammes)

Laboratory Investigations

The following procedure for specimens and their accompanying request forms is vital.

Specimen
Collect each specimen into the correct container and immediately label with the patient's full name, identifying particulars and date. A single forename and surname, as in 'Mary Jones', may not distinguish between two patients on the same ward. Any confusion, particularly concerning blood transfusion, can be fatal.

Send specimen to Laboratory without delay. Normally this should be early in the day.

Request for Investigation
An appropriate request form must accompany each specimen and provide the following information:
1. Patient's surname, forename, sex, age (or date of birth) and hospital registration number if available. The patient's address should also be given with all requests for blood grouping and cross-matching.
2. Hospital and ward; or address and telephone number of practice or clinic.
3. Nature of specimen with date and time of collection.
4. Examination required.
5. Provisional diagnosis and clinical summary, with stress on information relevant to the investigation.
6. Signature of clinician making request and date.
Requests should not be made by telephone except in dire emergency. In such emergency the patient's name must be spelt or lettered over the telephone. The telephone message must be confirmed by a request form (mandatory for blood transfusion requests).

Contents

SECTION ONE
The Alimentary System

The Alimentary System

ORAL CYTOLOGY

By taking cytological smears from abnormal lesions in the mouth, particularly in older people, it is possible to detect cancer at the very early stage when it can be readily treated. The material may be collected either by touching or by scraping.

1. *Touch preparation*. Where the situation allows, a glass slide may be applied directly to the surface of the lesion. A gentle touch suffices, repeated at different sites on the slide, or on different slides, and immediately fixed.

2. *Scrape and smear*. The surface of the lesion is gently scraped with a spatula and the material spread evenly on a slide, avoiding a rotary motion. With either method the material must be fixed while still moist and the slide be labelled immediately.

TEST FOR OESOPHAGITIS (Bernstein, Baker and Earlam)

The patient swallows a pernasal catheter until its tip is 30–35cm from the incisor teeth. Connected to the catheter by a Y-tube are two drip bottles with taps, one bottle containing normal saline (150mmol/litre), the other containing hydrochloric acid (100mmol/litre). Saline alone dripped into the oesophagus should cause no pain and acts as a control. Switching to the acid (6–7ml/min) causes pain if oesophagitis is present. Relief of the pain by sodium bicarbonate (100mmol/litre) is characteristic. This test distinguishes the pain of oesophagitis from other causes of chest pain.

OESOPHAGOSCOPY

This is the examination of the inner lining of the oesophagus by means of a special instrument called an oesophagoscope. It is a tube with a light at one end, which is introduced into the oesophagus through the mouth. Recently a flexible instrument has been introduced which is less uncomfortable for the patient than the rigid one. It is used for the investigation of growths and strictures of the oesophagus, the removal of accessible foreign bodies, also the collection of small portions of tissue for histological examination and material for cytology. The preparation and after-care of the patient are as described below for gastroscopy.

Gastric Investigations

Improved techniques have made it possible to examine the stomach with greater precision. These techniques include double-contrast radiography, gastroscopy using a flexible fibre-optic endoscope, multiple biopsies, brushing cytology and photography. By their use gastric cancer is being diagnosed at a curable stage with increasing frequency in Japan and more recently in Europe and America.

For testing gastric secretion, Pentagastrin has now become the method of choice (p. 15), apart from Insulin stimulation (Hollander test, p. 17) which is used to check whether the operation of 'highly selective vagotomy' has been successful. Gruel, alcohol and histamine test meals are now little used.

DOUBLE CONTRAST RADIOGRAPHY

A double contrast x-ray is obtained by introducing gas and barium into the stomach. It enables much smaller abnormalities to be demonstrated than with the ordinary barium meal (p. 209).

GASTROSCOPY

By means of a gastroscope the interior of the stomach may be examined visually, material taken for histological and

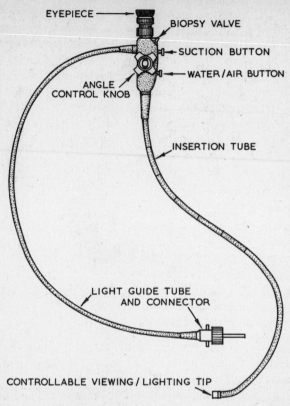

EYEPIECE

BIOPSY VALVE

SUCTION BUTTON

WATER/AIR BUTTON

ANGLE
CONTROL KNOB

INSERTION TUBE

LIGHT GUIDE TUBE
AND CONNECTOR

CONTROLLABLE VIEWING/LIGHTING TIP

Fig. 1/1   Flexible fibre-optic gastroscope

cytological diagnosis, abnormalities photographed and a
sketch made of the findings and of biopsy sites. The fibre-
optic gastroscope (endoscope) consists of a firm but flexible
plastic tube with a controllable end bearing a light (Fig.
1/1). It is passed into the stomach through the mouth and
oesophagus (Fig. 1/2). A bundle of finely drawn glass fibres
(the fibre optics) passing through the tube connects the
eyepiece to the flexible tip, enabling the lining membrane
of the stomach to be examined. The examination is often

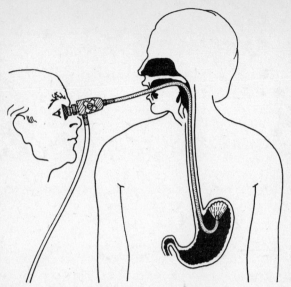

Fig. 1/2   Gastroscope introduced into the stomach with tip flexed to examine the fundus

carried out in the morning, with the patient in a fasting condition, nothing having been taken since midnight. If gastroscopy is to be undertaken in the afternoon, the patient fasts after having a light breakfast of tea and toast at 06.00h. One hour before the examination diazepam (Valium) 10mg is given. Fifteen minutes before gastroscopy a tablet of amethocaine is given, followed by a second tablet as the patient is taken to the theatre.

In skilled hands the passage of the gastroscope into the stomach should cause relatively little discomfort. During the gastroscopy multiple photographs are often taken, e.g. of an ulcer or growth. A sketch is also made on which the numbered biopsy sites are marked. Material for cytology is collected by means of a gastroscopy brush with a protective plastic tube to prevent carry-over of cells from one case to the next. Alternatively the whole gastroscope may be withdrawn with the brush still protruding. Material from the brush is immediately smeared evenly on to two to four microscope slides, spray-fixed while still moist and the slides labelled.

Following the examination, mucus and air may be brought up. Owing to the local anaesthetic, nothing should be allowed by mouth for 1 to 2 hours, as fluid may be inhaled into the lungs. If the throat is sore following the examination, a simple inhalation may be given.

Gastroscopy is of assistance in the diagnosis of gastritis, gastric and duodenal ulcers, and carcinoma of the stomach. Atrophy of the mucosa is seen in cases of pernicious anaemia and with other gastric lesions.

GASTROCAMERA EXAMINATION

The gastrocamera is introduced into the stomach in the same way as a gastroscope, which it resembles, but it has a tiny camera at its tip, enabling high quality pictures of the gastric mucosa to be taken directly instead of through the fibre optics of a gastroscope, giving better definition.

PENTAGASTRIN 'TEST MEAL'

Pentagastrin is chemically similar to the normal gastric stimulant hormone gastrin, and has now virtually replaced alcohol, histamine and the gruel test meal. The patient is allowed no food or drink after midnight. At 06.00h a Ryle's tube is passed pernasally into the stomach; a mark on the tube shows when it has passed far enough. Resting juice is collected at 15-minute intervals for a period of 1 hour to determine the basal acid output (BAO). Pentagastrin (Peptavlon) is then injected subcutaneously in a dose of $6\mu g/kg$ body-weight using a tuberculin syringe. Specimens are collected at 15-minute intervals, usually for a further period of 1 hour. The volume of each sample is measured and it is then filtered through gauze into a bottle. The acidity is estimated in the laboratory. The peak acid output

(PAO) is 2 × (the sum of the two consecutive 15-minute acid outputs giving the largest total). A normal example is shown in Figure 1/3.

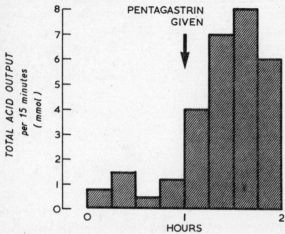

Fig. 1/3   Pentagastrin 'test meal'

Interpretation:	BAO (mmol/h)	PAO (mmol/h)
Normal subjects	1–8	1–50
Gastric cancer	0–8	0–30
Gastric ulcer	0–8	1–50
Duodenal ulcer	0–25	15–100
Pernicious anaemia	0	0
Zollinger–Ellison syndrome	over 15	15–100
(See Gastrin p. 18)		

The success of the test depends on good collections of gastric juice. If these are incomplete the test is valueless. The absence of acid in pernicious anaemia may be confirmed by pH measurement which remains at about pH 7 (see p. 100).

INSULIN 'TEST MEAL' (Hollander test)

The fasting patient is intubated as for the Pentagastrin 'test meal'. The fasting juice is aspirated and discarded. The basal secretion is collected over the next two 30-minute periods. Soluble insulin 15–20 units is then given intravenously. Gastric juice is collected for a further four 30-minute periods. Blood is taken at 30 and 45 minutes after the insulin injection into fluoride tubes for glucose estimation. All the specimens are sent to the laboratory for analysis of volume, and free and total acid secretion.

Insulin stimulation tests the integrity of the vagus nerve and is usually carried out about 1 week after the operation of 'highly selective vagotomy'. The insulin produces a low blood sugar (hypoglycaemia) which causes the vagus nerve to promote the secretion of acid and gastrin. This response is abolished if the operation has been successful.

ALCOHOL AND HISTAMINE 'TEST MEALS'

The patient is prepared as for the Pentagastrin 'test meal' (p. 15), and the resting juice similarly collected. The patient then drinks 50–100ml of 7% ethyl alcohol. Specimens of gastric juice are collected quarter hourly. At the end of 1 hour the patient may be given an injection of histamine hydrochloride 0.25–0.5mg subcutaneously. This is a powerful stimulant of gastric secretion. Further specimens of gastric juice are collected half and one hour after the histamine injection. If no free acid is detected in the latter specimens, the patient has histamine-fast achlorhydria, a typical finding in pernicious anaemia. Alternatively, the alcohol may be omitted, the patient being given histamine only, i.e. the Histamine 'Test Meal'. The 'augmented histamine test meal' in which the patient was protected from side-effects of the extra large dose of histamine by an antihistamine drug is no longer used. Most hospitals now use the Pentagastrin 'test meal' instead of any of the above.

GASTRIN

This hormone, produced by G cells of the gastric antrum and the duodenum, stimulates gastric secretion. Its normal range in the plasma is 5–50pmol/litre. Patients with a gastrin-producing tumour (Zollinger–Ellison or ZE syndrome) usually have over 100pmol/litre. However, patients with hypochlorhydria may have over 1000pmol/litre. So a high plasma gastrin only indicates ZE syndrome if there is also a high gastric acid. Collect 8ml blood into heparin tubes and transport immediately to the laboratory.

TESTS FOR MALABSORPTION OF VITAMIN B_{12}

Normal gastric juice contains intrinsic factor which is essential for the absorption of vitamin B_{12}. In pernicious anaemia intrinsic factor is absent so that vitamin B_{12} cannot be absorbed. Its absorption may also be impaired by defective intestinal mucosa as in intestinal malabsorption.

1. Schilling test
A small dose of radioactive B_{12} is given by mouth to the fasting patient, followed by a large dose (e.g. $1000\mu g$) of non-radioactive B_{12} intramuscularly. All urine for the next 24 hours is collected and sent to the laboratory. (**Note**. Complete urine collection is vital.) Normally more than 7 per cent of the radioactive dose is excreted in the urine in 24 hours. In pernicious anaemia less than 3 per cent is excreted.

If less than 7 per cent of the dose is excreted in the urine the patient is given a capsule containing $60\mu g$ of intrinsic factor and the test repeated as before. If the amount of radioactive B_{12} excreted now reaches normal levels the diagnosis of pernicious anaemia is confirmed. Failure to reach normal levels after the intrinsic factor has been given indicates intestinal malabsorption.

2. Dicopac test
The pack for this test is produced by The Radiochemical

Centre (Amersham, England). It involves one administration by capsules, one injection and one urine collection. In principle it is similar to the Schilling test but in practice it is more convenient.

The above tests have the great advantage that they can be used for treated cases without suspension of treatment.

VITAMIN B_{12} ESTIMATION (see p. 251)

Liver Function Tests

The liver carries out many different chemical processes. In any particular liver condition only some of these may be affected. A number of different tests for liver function are therefore necessary. The routine tests on urine and blood will first be described.

i. Routine Urine Tests for Liver Function (ward or clinic tests)

1. BILE PIGMENTS (BILIRUBIN)

Yellow froth on the urine when it is shaken suggests bilirubin. A test for bilirubin in urine is the Ictotest which may be done on the ward. Five drops of urine are placed on one square of the test mat provided. An Ictotest tablet is put in the centre of the moist area. Two drops of water are allowed to flow on to the tablet. The mat turns bluish-purple within 30 seconds if bilirubin is present. The speed and intensity of the colour is proportional to the amount of bilirubin. If no bilirubin is present the mat may turn pink, red or remain unchanged. (A more convenient test is Bililabstix, p. 152.)

2. UROBILIN

To 10ml of urine 1ml of Ehrlich's aldehyde reagent is added. After 3–5 minutes normal urine shows a faint reddish tinge, intensified by heating. If urobilin is increased a red colour is given by the urine, even diluted with about five times its own volume of water.

ii. Routine Blood Tests for Liver Function

10ml of blood in a plain sterile container is normally sufficient for all the following tests to be performed by the biochemistry department of most laboratories.

1. SERUM BILIRUBIN

This is estimated by the Van den Bergh test. Normally it is less than 20μmol/litre (1.2mg/100ml). When bilirubin has passed through the liver cells it is altered (conjugated) and gives a direct Van den Bergh reaction. In obstructive jaundice it regurgitates back into the blood, producing an increase in the conjugated (direct) serum bilirubin. In haemolytic jaundice excessive breakdown of red cells causes increased production of the bilirubin which has not passed through the liver cells and so is unconjugated, giving an indirect Van den Bergh reaction.

2. SERUM ALKALINE PHOSPHATASE (see p. 83)

Normally it is 10–40iu/litre (3–13 King Armstrong units) with higher values in infancy, childhood and also in pregnancy.

3. SERUM AMINOTRANSFERASES (TRANSAMINASES) (see p. 91)

Normally there are up to 35iu/litre of each aminotransferase, i.e. AST (SGOT) and ALT (SGPT).

4. SERUM GAMMA-GLUTAMYL TRANSFERASE (TRANSPEPTIDASE), γ GT

The normal range is 10–45iu/litre in men and 10–35iu/litre in women (see p. 93).

5. PROTEINS AND ELECTROPHORESIS (see p. 98)

Normally about 70g/litre (7g/100ml) of protein is present in the serum, of which 45g/litre (4.5g/100ml) are albumin and 25g/litre (2.5g/100ml) globulin.

Interpretation of Routine Liver Function Tests

When liver function is sufficiently impaired to interfere with the excretion of bile pigments, jaundice results. It is due to the retention of the bile pigment bilirubin in the blood. (Bilirubin is formed from the breakdown of haemoglobin from destroyed red blood cells.)

Jaundice may be of three types:

1. *Obstructive,* due to blockage of the bile ducts, e.g. by gall stones.
2. *Haemolytic*, due to excessive destruction of the red blood cells, e.g. acholuric jaundice.
3. *Toxic or infective*, due to chemical or inflammatory damage to the liver cells, e.g. infective hepatitis.

Typical results in the different types of jaundice:

1. OBSTRUCTIVE JAUNDICE

Urine: Bile salts and pigments present.
      Urobilin absent.
Blood: Bilirubin. Increased direct (conjugated).
      Alkaline phosphatase. Much increased.
      Aminotransferases. Often normal but sometimes increased, ALT (SGPT) often more than AST (SGOT) (see p. 91).
      γ GT. Normal or slightly increased (see p. 93).
      Proteins. Normal.

2. HAEMOLYTIC JAUNDICE, E.G. ACHOLURIC JAUNDICE

Urine: Bile salts and pigments absent.
      Urobilin. Increased, often greatly.
Blood: Bilirubin increased (indirect or unconjugated).
      Aminotransferases (AST and ALT) only
      increased in 50 per cent of cases. Other liver
      function tests normal.

3. TOXIC AND INFECTIVE HEPATITIS

Urine: Bile salts and pigments present.
      Urobilin. Variable.
Blood: Bilirubin increased, usually mainly direct (conju-
      gated).
      Alkaline phosphatase. Increased.
      Aminotransferases. Greatly increased, especially
      ALT (SGPT).
      γ GT. Greatly increased.
      Proteins. Albumin diminished.
      Globulin increased.
      The ratio may be reversed.
      Iron. Increased (see p. 95).

Additional Liver Function Tests

INTRAVENOUS DYE TEST (BROMSULPHALEIN OR BSP TEST)

A special dye, usually Bromsulphalein (BSP or sulpho-
bromophthalein sodium), is injected intravenously. The
dye is put up in ampoules, and the amount used depends on
the weight of the patient (5mg/kg). At 30 and 45 minutes
after injection, using fresh syringes, 5–10ml samples of
blood are collected and sent to the laboratory. Normally
less than 15 per cent of the dye remains after 30 minutes

and less than 5 per cent after 45 minutes. With liver damage the dye is not excreted normally and more dye remains in the blood, e.g. up to 50 per cent at 45 minutes in cirrhosis.

HIPPURIC ACID TEST (oral method)

The patient is given a light breakfast 2–3 hours before the test. Then 6g of sodium benzoate in 30ml of water, followed by half a tumbler of water. The bladder is immediately emptied completely and the urine thrown away.

Hourly specimens of urine are collected for the next 4 hours and all the urine sent to the laboratory. Normally at least 3.5g of hippuric acid (expressed as sodium benzoate) is excreted in the 4 hours. This is reduced in liver damage.

The test is not reliable if kidney disease is present or if absorption is impaired. An intravenous method can be used to overcome poor absorption, but the hippuric acid test is now seldom used.

SERUM IRON (see p. 95)

Normal serum iron is 1–3mmol/litre (60–180μg/ml). This is increased in toxic and infective liver disease, with values over 3.5mmol/litre (210μg/ml). It may help to distinguish them from jaundice due to mechanical obstruction where values below 3.5mmol/litre are obtained.

SERUM CHOLESTEROL (see p. 84)

INVESTIGATION OF DUODENAL CONTENTS FOR BILE SECRETION (see Duodenal Aspiration Tests, p. 26)

ERCP (Endoscopic Retrograde Cholangio-Pancreatography, see p. 27)

LIVER PUNCTURE BIOPSY

This test enables liver tissue to be obtained for histological examination without the dangers of a laparotomy and anaesthesia. Before the test is performed, bleeding, clotting, prothrombin times and platelet count must be determined, in order to exclude any bleeding tendency. Vitamin K (e.g. Synkavit) may be given if the prothrombin time is prolonged.

The patient's blood must be grouped and suitable blood made available for cross-match. Liver function tests should also be carried out. Half an hour before the puncture a mild sedative may be given if required, e.g. diazepam (Valium) 5–10mg. Stronger narcosis prevents the patient from cooperating.

A sterile trolley is prepared containing towels, swabs, skin cleansing materials, 2% lignocaine hydrochloride solution with syringe and needles, tenotomy knife, and special liver puncture biopsy set, including 20ml syringe to fit where required. Collodion dressing should be on the trolley, also specimen containers, viz one containing absolute alcohol (or Masson's fixative), one containing formal saline, and a dry sterile container, useful for cryostat work or for culture.

The patient lies on his back on his bed, his right hand under his head and his side parallel with the edge of the bed. He is told that he must follow the doctor's instructions regarding breathing while the puncture is being performed. By means of the special puncture needle a small cylinder of liver tissue is removed. This is either placed immediately in fixative or else taken unfixed direct to the laboratory for frozen section. Following the puncture careful watch must be kept on the pulse rate and blood pressure for any sign of internal haemorrhage. They must be recorded every 15 minutes for the first 2 hours and then hourly for the next 22 hours, any rise in the pulse rate or fall in blood pressure being notified to the physician at once.

By this procedure many conditions can be diagnosed, including cirrhosis of the liver, neoplasms, amyloidosis and miliary tuberculosis. See also biopsy (p. 242).

Pancreatic Efficiency Tests

The pancreas has two separate functions.
1. The secretion of pancreatic juice into the small intestine.
2. The secretion of insulin into the bloodstream.

Tests Related to the Secretion of Pancreatic Juice

1. EXAMINATION OF STOOLS

a. Trypsin test (suitable only for children)
A sample of fresh faeces is sent to the laboratory where the presence and concentration of trypsin is detected by its ability to digest protein (e.g. gelatin or an exposed x-ray film).

b. Fat in stools (p. 35)
This is estimated in the laboratory. Increased unsplit fat in the stools suggests pancreatic disease, but normal fat does not exclude the condition.

c. Muscle fibres in stools
A marked increase in the number of undigested muscle fibres in the stools may occur in pancreatic disease but is not constant.

2. TESTS FOR PANCREATITIS

a. Serum Amylase (or Diastase)
About 5ml of fresh clotted blood should be sent to the laboratory. Normally the serum amylase is 90–270iu/litre (60–180 Somogyi units/100 ml). In acute pancreatitis it rises greatly soon after the onset, over 1200iu/litre units being considered diagnostic. But it may return to normal limits in a few days even though the disease is not subsiding. A slight rise may occur in chronic pancreatitis.

b. Urine Amylase (or Diastase)

If urgent a single urine specimen will suffice. Otherwise a 24-hour specimen should be collected, preserved with a little toluene. Normally urine amylase is 130–1 300iu/litre (5–50 Wohlgemuth units). Levels of 25 000iu/litre (1 000 Wohlgemuth units) or more may be reached in acute pancreatitis, falling to normal slightly later than the serum amylase.

3. DUODENAL ASPIRATION TESTS

These necessitate the passage of a special tube into the duodenum. The tube has a double lumen, one opening into the duodenum and the other into the stomach. Preparation of the patient is similar to that for the Pentagastrin 'test meal' (p. 15). The tests are most conveniently performed under fluoroscopic control. The patient then sits with the tube in position while continuous suction at a controlled pressure (25–40mmHg) is applied to the duodenum for 80 minutes. Suction is also applied to the mouth and stomach to remove saliva and gastric juice.

Pancreatic Secretion (Secretin Test)
Pancreatic secretion is stimulated by secretin. (An injection of 1 clinical unit per kilogram body-weight of secretin from the GIH Research Unit of the Karolinska Institute gives maximal stimulation.) The aspirated fluid from the duodenum is collected into ice-cooled flasks containing an equal quantity of glycerol. In pancreatic disease, the enzymes are reduced, particularly amylase. Pancreozymin injection is sometimes given as a more specific stimulus of enzyme secretion. In more severe conditions bicarbonate is also reduced. Some workers now consider that bicarbonate estimation is the best guide to pancreatic exocrine function.

Lundh Test
Instead of using secretin, a special test meal is given to stimulate pancreatic secretion. It consists of milk powder, vegetable oil and dextrose. Fluid from the proximal jejunum is aspirated over the next 2 hours and the mean trypsin level estimated. This test is simpler to perform than the secretin test but less accurate.

Secretion of Bile

Absence of bile from all specimens indicates bile duct obstruction. Stimulation of bile secretion by 25% magnesium sulphate at 37°C injected through the duodenal tube is occasionally used. Pus cells are found in cholecystitis. The causative organism may be obtained on culture. Typhoid bacilli have occasionally been isolated from 'carriers'. (See also Vi test, p. 74.)

4. ERCP (Endoscopic Retrograde Cholangio-Pancreatography)

Using a duodenoscope (a larger version of the gastroscope) it is possible to introduce a tube into the ampulla of Vater, under fluoroscopy. Preparation of the patient is similar to that for gastroscopy. Specimens may be collected for chemistry and cytology (for the diagnosis of pancreatic cancer). A radio-opaque medium is then injected to outline the pancreatic duct and the biliary tract, e.g. to demonstrate the site of a tumour.

5. SWEAT TEST

In children with fibrocystic disease the sodium chloride content of sweat is increased. This may be detected as follows. Sweating is stimulated, usually on the forearm, or in babies on the thigh, by means of a pad moistened with pilocarpine solution (e.g. 0.2% pilocarpine nitrate in distilled water) through which a mild electric current is passed for 5 minutes, using an iontophoresis apparatus. The stimulated area is washed with distilled water and dried. An accurately weighed filter paper is placed on the prepared area and covered by a slightly larger polythene sheet which is strapped into position for half an hour. The filter paper is returned to its original container and sent without delay to the laboratory where the sweat is analysed. In fibrocystic disease the sodium level is increased, usually above 60mmol/litre (60mEq/litre).

Tests Related to Insulin Secretion

1. SUGAR IN URINE

a. Clinitest
Five drops of urine are placed in a test-tube. The dropper is rinsed and ten drops of water added. One Clinitest tablet is dropped in and spontaneous boiling occurs. Fifteen seconds after the boiling stops the tube is shaken gently and compared with the Clinitest colour scale to estimate the amount of sugar present.

b. Benedict's test
Eight drops of urine are added to 5ml of Benedict's solution in a test-tube and boiled for 5 minutes. If sugar is present the colour changes and is estimated by the degree of change. Viz Green = a trace. Yellow = +. Orange = + +. Brick red = + + +.

c. Clinistix
The test end of a Clinistix, dipped into the urine and removed, should change colour in 10 seconds if glucose is present. Laboratory confirmation is essential. Patients receiving large doses of vitamin C may give false negative results.

2. KETONES IN URINE

a. Acetest
An Acetest tablet is placed on a clean white surface. One drop of urine is put on the tablet. After 30 seconds the colour is compared with the Acetest colour scale. The test detects acetone and acetoacetic acid. A moderate or strongly positive result indicates a severe ketosis.

b. Ketostix
This stick test is simpler to perform than the above: the end of the stick is dipped into the urine and read after 15 seconds. Its interpretation is similar to the Acetest (a).

c. Rothera's test

To 10ml of urine in a test-tube add sufficient ammonium sulphate crystals to make a saturated solution, add three drops of freshly prepared sodium nitroprusside solution and 2ml of strong ammonia. A purple colour forms at the junction of the two liquids if ketone bodies are present. (A very sensitive test.)

d. Gerhardt's test

About 5ml of urine are put in a test-tube, and 10% ferric chloride solution added drop by drop. At first a white precipitate forms which disappears on adding more ferric chloride. A port wine colour develops if acetoacetic acid is present. A false positive result may be given if the patient has been taking certain drugs, e.g. aspirin. If tests (c) and (d) are positive in the absence of drugs, the patient has severe ketosis, as in diabetes and severe starvation.

3. BLOOD SUGAR (preferably fasting) (see p. 102)

4. GLUCOSE TOLERANCE TESTS

a. Glucose Tolerance Test

This test measures the patient's ability to stabilise his blood sugar level after taking a quantity of glucose. The absorption of glucose raises the blood sugar level and the action of insulin lowers it.

The test is done in the morning, the patient having fasted since 22.00h the previous evening (water may be drunk). A specimen of blood is taken for the fasting sugar estimation and the bladder emptied. The patient is given 75g of glucose dissolved in about 300ml of water to drink, flavoured with diabetic squash. For children, a smaller quantity of glucose is given (1.75g/kg body-weight). Further specimens of blood are taken for blood sugar estimation after $\frac{1}{2}$ hour, 1 hour, 1$\frac{1}{2}$ hours and 2 hours, and corresponding specimens of urine are collected.

Typical results of the test are shown in Figure 1/4. In

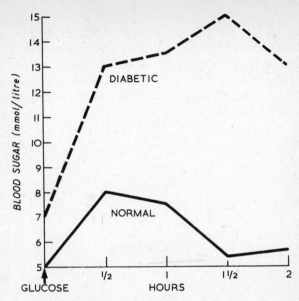

Fig. 1/4   Glucose tolerance test

normal persons the blood sugar resumes its normal level of about 5.6mmol/litre (100mg/100ml) within 2 hours. Diagnostic values for diabetes are a fasting whole blood level of at least 7.0mmol/litre and/or a level of at least 10.0mmol/litre at 2h after the glucose. Corresponding plasma levels are 8.0mmol/litre and 11.0mmol/litre. In the malabsorption syndrome the glucose is only absorbed slowly, so that a 'flat curve' is produced.

b. Extended Glucose Tolerance Test

If hypoglycaemia is suspected, e.g. in a child having fits, it is usually necessary to extend the test to 5 hours. For convenience blood sugar estimations up to 4 hours may be omitted. In spontaneous hypoglycaemia the blood sugar may fall to a very low level towards the end of the test, e.g. below 3.6mmol/litre (65mg/100ml).

5. SERUM INSULIN

This assay is only indicated for the differential diagnosis of hypoglycaemia after this has been confirmed by accurate blood glucose analysis. In normal people fasting induces hypoglycaemia with a low serum insulin. Insulin levels are usually above 10mU/litre in cases of insulinoma, however low the blood glucose. On each of three successive mornings after a 15-hour fast (18.00h to 09.00h) two samples of blood are collected: 2ml into a fluoride tube for glucose and 5ml clotted blood for insulin. These are sent at once to the laboratory. During the fast the patient may drink tap water. If symptoms of hypoglycaemia occur blood samples must be collected before giving food.

When the results are equivocal the diagnosis of insulinoma is supported if the serum insulin remains above 4mU/litre when the blood glucose is reduced below 3mmol/litre (54mg/100ml) by the injection of fish insulin. The laboratory will give details of an alternative (porcine insulin) test.

6. PLASMA GLUCAGON

Its estimation is only of value in the pre-operative diagnosis of a glucagon producing tumour of the pancreas, characterised by wasting diabetes, anaemia and skin rash (necrolytic migratory erythema). Normally fasting levels are always below 100ng/litre. Glucagonomas produce levels of up to 1 000ng/litre or more. Details of this specialised SAS investigation can be obtained from the laboratory.

BIOPSY OF THE SMALL INTESTINE

By means of an instrument such as the Crosby capsule it is possible to obtain a specimen of tissue from the small intestine for examination. The capsule contains a guarded cutting mechanism actuated via a long thin flexible tube. It is usually swallowed in the morning, the patient having

fasted since midnight. From the stomach it gradually pro-
gresses through the duodenum to the jejunum, which it
reaches in about an hour or two, the patient lying on his
right side. The position of the capsule is checked by x-ray
and the biopsy taken from the appropriate site by applying
suction to the tube. It is used in the investigation of coeliac
disease (see p. 35).

ASCITIC FLUID

Ascites is the accumulation of fluid (ascitic fluid) in the
peritoneal cavity. It occurs in failure of the liver, heart and
kidneys and in abdominal tumours and inflammations. It is
obtained by paracentesis, i.e. the aseptic introduction into
the peritoneal cavity of a sterile aspiration needle or a
trocar and cannula. Often sterile plastic tubing is introduced through the cannula to facilitate subsequent drainage, the rate of drainage being controlled by a clip. Samples
of fluid are collected and examined. The fluid may be
examined for the types of cell present (p. 246), organisms
(p. 229) and chylomicrons, which are minute fat droplets
seen in thoracic duct lesions.

LAPAROSCOPY

This is the examination of the peritoneal cavity with a
laparoscope (a sort of telescope) through a small abdominal incision under local anaesthesia. It is used occasionally
for examination of the liver but more often in the investigation of lower abdominal pain which cannot be diagnosed
by other methods. It is also being used increasingly for
female sterilisation.

PROCTOSCOPY

This enables the anal canal and lower 8cm (3in) of the
rectum to be examined. It is preferable for the bowel to
have been emptied prior to the test. The patient is placed in

the left lateral, or knee–elbow position, as for a rectal examination. A warmed and lubricated proctoscope is passed. It is of value for the examination of haemorrhoids and growths, from which a specimen may be taken for biopsy.

SIGMOIDOSCOPY

The sigmoidoscope is a metal or plastic tube with electric illumination which enables the rectum and sigmoid colon to be examined. The examination may be carried out in the ward, outpatient clinic or operating theatre, without anaesthetic.

It is used in the differential diagnosis of ulcerative colitis, amoebic dysentery and growths.

COLONOSCOPY

The colonoscope consists of a long firm flexible plastic tube, with a controllable end bearing a light, with which it is possible to examine the entire length of the colon (Fig. 1/5). Vision is made possible by fibre optics, as in the flexible gastroscope (p. 13), but the colonoscope is much longer and the glass fibres are more easily damaged by bending. This limits the number of colonoscopies that can be undertaken before the instrument requires costly repair. Preparation of the patient involves a 3-day regime. On day 1, all constipating drugs are stopped, including oral iron, and a clear fluid diet is started. If the patient is constipated 2 Senokot tablets are given in the evening. On day 2, fluids only are continued. In the morning 1 litre of 10% mannitol in tap water is given, to be drunk over a period of 30–60 minutes. On day 3, no breakfast is given, fluids are continued and a rectal washout administered 2 hours before colonoscopy. As an alternative fluid-only regime the patient drinks 100ml sorbitol 70% followed by 500ml of water on the first morning. This is repeated 4 hours later and again on morning 2 followed by a rectal washout until clear, with a further rectal washout on day 3 prior to endoscopy. For very con-

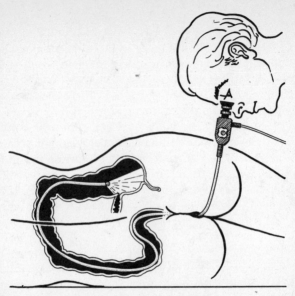

Fig. 1/5   Colonoscope introduced into the colon

stipated elderly patients the sorbitol regime may be started 2 days earlier. At 1 hour before the examination Valium 10 mg is usually prescribed.

Colonoscopy is best undertaken in a special room with a table on which the patient lies in the left lateral position. The colonoscope is introduced through the anus and its progress up the colon is monitored by x-ray. It may cause physical and/or psychological discomfort and the nurse can assist greatly by reassuring the patient. Colonoscopy is used mainly for investigating possible malignant change in the colon, e.g. in polyposis or chronic ulcerative colitis, and enables multiple biopsies to be taken for histology.

TESTS FOR INTESTINAL MALABSORPTION
(Malabsorption Syndromes)

1. D-Xylose Excretion Test
This is a convenient test for the malabsorption syndromes, e.g. coeliac disease. The fasting patient is given 5g of D-xylose sugar by mouth, dissolved in about 600ml water. All urine is collected for the next 5 hours and sent to the laboratory. Normally this contains more than 1g of xylose. If there is malabsorption it is diminished. With children the test is generally carried out using only $\frac{1}{3}$g/kg body-weight; of this $\frac{1}{5}$ of the dose should be found in the 5-hour urine specimen.

2. Glucose Tolerance Test (see p. 29)
Typically a 'flat curve' is obtained in intestinal malabsorption, due to slow absorption of the glucose.

3. Faecal Fat
Fat Balance. The patient is put on the normal ward diet which should contain 70g of fat per day. After a few days to allow stabilization, all the faeces are collected for an exact period of time, e.g. 3 or 5 days. To make the test more accurate a 'marker' dye may be given by mouth at the beginning and end of the 3- or 5-day period. With the appearance of the first 'marker' the faeces collection is started, and with the appearance of the second it is stopped. Normally the fat excreted does not exceed 5g/24h and at least 90 per cent of the fat taken is absorbed. Less than 90 per cent suggests malabsorption.

4. Tests for Malabsorption of Vitamin B_{12} (see p. 18)
Defective vitamin B_{12} absorption, indicated by the low urine excretion values, is not rectified by giving intrinsic factor.

5. Biopsy of the Small Intestine (see p. 31)
The mucosa shows flattening or absence of the villi in coeliac disease (gluten enteropathy, idiopathic steatorrhoea).

6. Bone Biopsy (see p. 244)

Malabsorption of vitamin D causes osteomalacia. This can be demonstrated by bone biopsy, with undecalcified sections to reveal the osteoid tissue.

Examination of the Faeces

OCCULT BLOOD TEST

Small quantities of blood in the stools can be detected by this test. The patient is given or advised to have a high residue diet for 3 days before the test and during the test period, avoiding any high dose vitamin C supplement during this time. The test now being used is Haemoccult. An outpatient is given three test envelopes with detailed easily understood directions for their use and applicators for taking samples of stool. On three consecutive days pea size samples are taken from two parts of the stool and spread on to the two red-framed openings inside the test envelope. If the patient does not have a bowel movement on one day the samples are taken from the next stool. The envelopes, with identity label completed, are sent to the laboratory at the end of the test.

In the laboratory the analyst opens the back of the envelope, involving no contact with the stool, and applies at least two drops of developer solution to each stool specimen site. A blue colour at 30 seconds is a positive test. One positive test from the six is a 'positive' result.

The occult blood test is of great value in gastric and duodenal ulcers, as an additional factor in diagnosis and also as a guide to whether the ulcer has healed or not. It is positive in an active ulcer and negative in a healed ulcer. It is usually continuously positive in cases of carcinoma of the stomach or in growths in any other part of the alimentary tract.

Much blood in the stools renders them black, but it should be borne in mind that black stools may be produced by the patient taking iron, bismuth or manganese.

FAT, MUSCLE FIBRES, TRYPSIN (see pancreatic efficiency tests, p. 25 and faecal fat, p. 35)

ORGANISMS AND PARASITES IN STOOLS

Numerous bacteria are present in normal stools. In typhoid, paratyphoid, dysentery and food poisoning the organisms carrying the disease are present in the stools. 'Carriers' have such organisms in their stools without having the disease, usually having recovered from it in the recent or distant past.

Where infection is suspected, a specimen of faeces is collected into the appropriate container for laboratory examination, with due precautions against spreading infection (e.g. on the hands or the outside of the container). Collection can be undertaken in an ordinary closet if, after micturition and flushing the pan, six pieces of newspaper are placed on the surface of the water before defaecation. Faecal material floating on the paper may then be transferred to the container using a wooden spatula. A negative culture does not exclude infection and at least three specimens should always be submitted. If amoebic dysentery is a possibility and the patient is in an acute phase, a specimen of faeces containing mucus should be sent to the laboratory while still warm. This greatly increases the chances of finding amoebae. In chronic cases and where intestinal parasites, e.g. tapeworms, roundworms or hookworms, are suspected, at least three specimens should be sent to the laboratory. Tubercle bacilli occur in the faeces of some cases of tuberculosis. In pseudomembranous colitis, Clostridium difficile or its toxin may be demonstrated. Enterocolitis, which can mimic an acute abdomen may be due to Yersinia enterocolitica. The Campylobacter species is another cause of diarrhoea or dysentery. Rotavirus can cause acute diarrhoea in infants up to 4 years old. The investigations for food-borne infection are described below.

Threadworm infestation may be demonstrated by swabbing the anal region with a bacteriological swab and sending it to the laboratory, clearly indicating the investigation required on the request form.

FOOD POISONING

This is almost always due to contamination of the food by organisms. The organisms most commonly found are those of the salmonella group, such as S. typhimurium and S. enteritidis (of Gaertner). Food poisoning is also commonly caused by Staphylococcus pyogenes which produces an exotoxin (enterotoxin), occasionally by Clostridium welchii and rarely by Clostridium botulinum. The organisms or their toxins may survive boiling for up to 20 minutes.

The following should be sent to the laboratory in suspected cases of food poisoning:

1. Portion of food suspected.
2. Stools (as soon as passed).
3. Vomited matter, or stomach contents from a gastric washout.
4. Blood, About 5ml in a dry sterile tube. Certain organisms give agglutination reactions similar to those given in the Widal test in typhoid fever (p. 73). These do not usually become positive until a week after infection.

NB The clinical history is of very great importance in establishing the diagnosis.

PORPHYRINS

Normally the faeces contain only traces of porphyrins (see p. 174) viz coproporphyrin < 30nmol (< 30μg) dry weight, protoporphyrin < 140nmol (< 140μg) dry weight. The increased amounts present in the porphyrias may be detected by laboratory screening tests.

SECTION TWO

Examination of the Blood

Part I. Haematology and Blood Transfusion

Part II. Bacteriological Tests on Blood

Part III. Chemical Tests on Blood

Examination of the Blood

Part I. Haematology and Blood Transfusion

This section deals with the tests concerning blood cells, bleeding and clotting, blood transfusion and other investigations performed in the haematology department.

BLOOD COUNTS

The tests most commonly needed are the haemoglobin (below), red cell appearance (p. 49) and white cell count (p. 50). These can all be undertaken on one 4ml sequestrenated sample of blood and are usually performed on automated equipment which provides seven separate results: haemoglobin, red cell count, white cell count, haematocrit (p. 47), and also the three main absolute values MCV, MCH and MCHC (p. 48). Platelet counts (p. 52) are also frequently required, especially to monitor drug toxicity. The other main investigations are the differential white cell count (p. 51) and the red cell appearance (p. 46).

HAEMOGLOBIN

Haemoglobin is a pigment in the red blood cells, which combines with oxygen to form a reversible compound (oxyhaemoglobin).

Estimation of the haemoglobin content of the blood is thus a measure of its oxygen-carrying capacity.

The average adult level is about 14.5g/dl (14.5g/100 ml) or 100 per cent. It is higher in men (12.5–18g/dl), and lower in women (11.5–16.5g/dl). At birth the cord blood haemoglobin is about 13.6–19.6g/dl, falling to about 12–15g/dl in the first few weeks of life.

In anaemia this figure is reduced below 11.5g/dl.

In polycythaemia it is increased to over 18g/dl.

It is also increased following fluid loss, e.g. from burns, vomiting, diarrhoea, diuresis or excessive sweating.

RED CELLS

The red cell count is normally about 5.00×10^{12}/litre (5 000 000 red cells per mm³) being slightly higher in males and lower in females.

The figure is decreased in anaemia and increased in polycythaemia. Dehydration from any cause, e.g. shock, vomiting, diarrhoea, excessive sweating or diuresis also causes a rise in the red cell count.

After haemorrhage it is about 24 hours before full reduction of the red cell count and haemoglobin can be demonstrated.

ERYTHROCYTE SEDIMENTATION RATE (ESR)

Normally the red blood cells do not show much tendency to aggregate on standing, with the result that sedimentation is slow. In certain diseases they run together very readily to form rouleaux which sediment more rapidly.

There are two common methods by which this test may be carried out, Wintrobe and Westergren. For the Wintrobe method, blood is collected into a Sequestrene bottle and sent to the laboratory without delay. The Westergren method is often performed in the ward and will therefore be described in more detail.

0.5ml of 3.8% sodium citrate is placed in a test-tube, to this is added 2ml of freshly taken blood and mixed. This mixture is then introduced into a graduated Westergren tube to the zero mark and the tube fixed into position on a special rack.

The distance fallen by the red blood cells is read at the end of 1 hour and sometimes after 2 hours. Normally it is 3–5mm in 1 hour for men and 4–7mm in 1 hour for women and children. It is of great value in estimating the progress in cases of tuberculosis, rheumatic fever and vasculitis.

It is raised in many other diseases, e.g. infections, infarctions and cancer, particularly in multiple myeloma. Anaemias generally cause a rise in the sedimentation rate, for which allowance must be made. With the Wintrobe method a correction factor may be applied and a result corrected for anaemia included in the report.

VISCOMETRY

This is the measurement of the viscosity of whole blood or plasma and is performed on sequestrenated blood. Blood viscosity is increased when there is increase in the PCV (see below). Plasma viscosity is increased when there is a raised ESR (see previous section). The increase is due to raised protein concentration, particularly fibrinogen. Some workers claim that plasma viscometry is a better test than the ESR, being quicker to perform.

HAEMATOCRIT (previously Packed Cell Volume or PCV)

As soon as possible after applying the tourniquet the appropriate volume of venous blood is collected into a container with anticoagulant (e.g. Sequestrene), mixed and sent to the laboratory. A representative portion is placed in a haematocrit tube and spun on a centrifuge until all the red cells are tightly packed at the bottom of the tube. Using automated equipment the haematocrit is a computed result based on the MCV and red cell count. The normal haematocrit is 0.35–0.54 (35–54 per cent) in men and 0.3–0.47 (30–47 per cent) in women. In anaemia it is reduced below these figures. It is increased in polycythaemia and dehydration. In the newborn the normal cord blood haematocrit is 0.44–0.62 (44–62 per cent).

It may be used to screen for anaemia, to indicate the degree of fluid loss, to correct the sedimentation rate for anaemia and to calculate certain absolute values (see below). With a microhaematocrit the test may be performed on a finger-prick sample.

'ABSOLUTE VALUES'

MCHC (Mean Cell Haemoglobin Concentration) indicates the degree to which cells are packed with haemoglobin. It is normally more than 30g/dl (30 per cent) and is reduced in iron deficiency. It is about the most reliable of the 'absolute values'.

MCD (Mean Cell Diameter) is the average diameter of the red cell, expressed in micrometres (μm). The average normal MCD is 7.2μm (normal range 6.7–7.7μm).

MCV (Mean Cell Volume) is the average volume of a single red cell, expressed in femtolitres (fl). Normally it is 86–100fl. In pernicious anaemia it is usually above 104fl.

MCH (Mean Cell Haemoglobin) is the average amount of haemoglobin in each red cell, normally 27–34pg.

Interpretation. In microcytic hypochromic anaemia, e.g. iron deficiency, all the absolute values are diminished.

In macrocytic anaemias, e.g. pernicious anaemia (PA) the absolute values are usually all raised with the exception of the MCHC which is either normal or reduced (if iron deficiency is also present).

RED CELL MASS

This test measures the total volume of all the circulating red cells. Blood is collected by the laboratory staff. The red cells are tagged with radioactive chromium, washed and re-injected into the patient. After 10 minutes blood is again collected. The haematocrit and radioactivity are measured. The red cell mass can then be calculated. Normally this is 30ml/kg for males and 27ml/kg for females. It is increased in polycythaemia, sometimes to more than twice the normal figure.

RETICULOCYTE COUNT

Very young red blood cells may be recognised by the fact that they take up a special stain that does not affect the mature red blood cells.

These young cells are called reticulocytes, because the stain demonstrates a network inside the cell (*reticulum* is Latin for a little net).

0.2 to 2 per cent reticulocytes are present in healthy people. A rise in the reticulocyte count is called a reticulocytosis and occurs as a response to satisfactory treatment in cases of anaemia. It also occurs following haemorrhage or haemolysis, due to the body's own power of regeneration.

On the routine blood film (e.g. stained with Leishman's stain) these young red cells have a bluish tinge described as polychromatic; so an increased number of polychromatic cells (called polychromasia) implies a reticulocytosis.

The 'stippling' of the red blood cells in lead poisoning is also associated with a reticulocytosis.

RED CELL APPEARANCE

On most haematological reports the appearance of the red cells, as seen on the stained film, is described. A cell of normal size is described as normocytic and one of normal colour as normochromic. Large cells, as seen for instance in pernicious anaemia, are called macrocytic, and small ones, as in iron deficiency, microcytic. Also in iron deficiency anaemia the cells are incompletely filled with haemoglobin giving them a pale appearance, described as hypochromic. Anisocytosis means excessive variation in size. Poikilocytosis means irregularity in shape.

PARASITES IN BLOOD

If a blood film is taken during an attack of malaria the parasites can be seen in the red blood cells. The best time for blood to be collected is about 2 hours after the temperature peak. The disease may recur several years after the original infection, especially with benign tertian malaria. If a fever occurs in a person who has been in districts where the anopheline mosquito breeds, a blood film should be taken. Latent malaria may be activated by some other disease, e.g. pneumonia, in which case there is a double diagnosis.

Blood parasites are found in other tropical diseases, e.g. trypanosomes in sleeping sickness, and spirochaetes in relapsing fever.

WHITE CELLS

The normal range of the white cell count is $4.0-11.0\times10^9$/litre ($4\,000-11\,000$/mm^3).

An increase above 11.0×10^9/litre is known as a leucocytosis. This occurs in infections, e.g. pneumonia, appendicitis, etc. A low figure in such conditions indicates a poor resistance on the part of the patient.

A great increase occurs in most types of leukaemia, especially in chronic myeloid leukaemia, sometimes up to 50.0×10^9/litre or more.

A decrease in the number below 4.0×10^9/litre is known as a leucopenia. It occurs in typhoid fever and aplastic anaemia; drugs, poisons and irradiation are important causes of leucopenia. An occasional cause is a leucocyte antibody. To detect this a special blood sample is collected by the laboratory.

Persons exposed continuously to x-rays, radium or other forms of radioactivity and certain industrial workers should have regular blood counts. Most people, if exposed excessively, first show an increase in the red cell count, followed later by a fall in the white cell count, and still later by an anaemia.

DIFFERENTIAL WHITE CELL COUNT

There are several different types of white cells, and the proportion of each type differs in various diseases. The differential count is carried out by microscopical examination of a stained film of blood on a glass slide.

Normal figures are:

Polymorphs $1.5–7.5×10^9$/litre (1 500–7 500 per mm³)
Lymphocytes $1.0–4.5×10^9$/litre (1 000–4 500 per mm³)
Monocytes   up to $0.8×10^9$/litre (800 per mm³)
Eosinophils   up to $0.4×10^9$/litre (400 per mm³)
Basophils   up to $0.2×10^9$/litre (200 per mm³)

To convert the percentage figures to the absolute figures as given above, the percentage figure for each type of cell is multiplied by the total white cell count, e.g.

Total white blood cells $10.0×10^9$/litre
Polymorphs 60 per cent
$$\therefore \frac{60}{100} \times 10.0 = 6.0 \times 10^9/\text{litre}$$

In most acute infections and in sepsis the polymorphs are increased. In glandular fever the lymphocytes and monocytes are increased. The eosinophils are increased in allergic conditions, e.g. asthma. In leukaemia abnormal cells of a primitive type are seen in the differential count.

A reduced polymorph (neutrophil) count is called a neutropenia. If polymorphs are less than 1.0×10^9/litre it is often called an agranulocytosis, most cases being the result of drugs or x-rays damaging the bone marrow.

BONE MARROW PUNCTURE

Examination of the bone marrow is an important part in the investigation of obscure anaemias.

The sites in which this is usually performed are the iliac crests and the sternum. In the obese the vertebral spines may be used.

A sterile trolley is required providing: dressing towels, skin antiseptic, swabs, 2% procaine hydrochloride with syringe and needles, and a tenotomy knife or small scalpel. The special marrow puncture needle, together with syringe to fit, are usually provided by the laboratory.

Marrow is aspirated from the bone cavity with full aseptic precautions, and spread on slides.

This procedure confirms the diagnosis in pernicious anaemia, leukaemia, multiple myeloma and other blood disorders.

Investigations for Haemorrhagic Disorders

ROUTINE BLOOD EXAMINATION (Haemoglobin, White Cell Count and Blood Film)

This may reveal that a bleeding disorder is due to a blood disease such as leukaemia or a platelet abnormality. The findings may indicate the need for a bone marrow puncture.

PLATELET COUNT

Blood platelets are normally present in the blood to the number of $150–350 \times 10^9$/litre (150 000–350 000 per mm^3).

Their chief function is to take part in the process of clotting of blood. Reduction of the platelets below a level of 40×10^9/litre is liable to be followed by haemorrhage.

Blood for this test is usually collected by the laboratory, but a Sequestrene sample is very satisfactory.

Platelets are diminished in thrombocytopenic purpura, PA, aplastic anaemia, acute leukaemia and other conditions, including auto-immune disease with platelet antibody formation. For detection of the latter, blood is collected by the laboratory staff.

The platelet count is not altered in haemophilia. Platelets are increased following operation, especially splenectomy, which may predispose towards thrombosis.

CAPILLARY RESISTANCE TEST (Hess's test)

A circle 6cm in diameter is marked out on the antecubital fossa. It is carefully examined under a bright light for any skin blemishes. A sphygmomanometer cuff is placed round the arm at least 3cm above the circle. A pressure of 50mmHg is maintained accurately for 15 minutes. After release the number of small haemorrhages (petechiae) appearing in the circle is counted. Up to eight is normal. It is increased when there is increased capillary fragility, e.g. in thrombocytopenic purpura.

BLEEDING TIME (Ivy's method)

Three small puncture wounds are made on the anterior aspect of the forearm, after a sphygmomanometer cuff has been applied and the pressure set at 40mmHg. The bleeding points are blotted at $\frac{1}{2}$-minute intervals, and the average time taken for two of the punctures to stop bleeding is taken.

Normal bleeding time is 3–5 minutes. It is prolonged in purpura, acute leukaemia, severe pernicious anaemia, and certain abnormalities of the blood vessels. It is normal in haemophilia.

CLOTTING TIME (Method of Lee and White)

One millilitre of blood is placed in each of four dry tubes, 0.6cm in diameter, stood in a water bath at 37°C. The clotting time is estimated as the average time taken for the first three tubes to clot.

The normal is 4–7 minutes. It is prolonged in haemophilia, Christmas disease, obstructive jaundice and during heparin treatment.

RECALCIFICATION TIME

This is the time taken for a fibrin clot to appear after the addition of calcium to plasma. It is more sensitive to slight disorder than the Clotting Time. Normally it is 90–125 seconds. It is increased in most coagulation disorders, e.g. haemophilia, Christmas disease, etc. Blood is collected by the laboratory technician.

CLOT RETRACTION

When blood has clotted the clot retracts, so that after 1 hour at 37°C normally 42–62 per cent of the original blood volume is serum. If platelets or fibrinogen are deficient it may fail to retract normally and show increased friability. Blood is collected by the laboratory technician.

PROTHROMBIN RATIO (Quick's One-stage Test)

Prothrombin is essential for blood clotting when it is converted into thrombin. This in turn converts fibrinogen into fibrin. Prothrombin cannot yet be estimated chemically. It is measured indirectly by the time taken for citrated plasma to clot after it has been activated. This is called the prothrombin time.

If the prothrombin time of a patient's plasma is twice as long as that of normal plasma, this is expressed as a prothrombin ratio of 2.0. The prothrombin index in this example would be 50 per cent, but this term is being abandoned in favour of prothrombin ratio (to avoid confusion with prothrombin activity which is also expressed as a percentage).

In the treatment of thrombo-phlebitis and allied disorders by anticoagulants the drugs should be adjusted to maintain the prothrombin ratio at 1.9 to 2.3. If the ratio increases much above this level there is a danger of haemorrhage.

The estimation is done by the laboratory on blood collected in a fresh citrate tube, usually specially provided for the purpose, particular care being taken to add the right amount of blood and mix well. It is also of value in investigating haemorrhagic disorders and liver disease.

There used to be considerable variation in the prothrombin ratio results between one hospital and another. By using a standardised reagent (Manchester Comparative Reagent) comparable results are produced at most British hospitals, the standardised ratio being expressed as the British Corrected Ratio (BCR).

TWO-STAGE PROTHROMBIN TEST

This is designed to estimate prothrombin more specifically than the preceding test. Normally prothrombin is 100 per cent. The figure is reduced in prothrombin deficiency and also by prothrombin inhibitor occurring in some cases of disseminated lupus erythematosus (DLE).

PROTHROMBIN AND PROCONVERTIN TEST

This differs from the Quick's one-stage prothrombin test in that fibrinogen and factor V are added, making it more sensitive to changes in factor VII, factor X and prothrombin (all of which depend on vitamin K for their formation). The specimen is collected by the laboratory technician. It can be performed on capillary plasma, a great advantage in small children. The normal range is 70–130 per cent. It forms the basis of the Thrombotest.

THROMBOTEST

This may be used instead of the prothrombin ratio to control anticoagulant therapy. The test may be carried out directly on finger-prick blood, thus avoiding venepuncture. The therapeutic level is 10–20 per cent, normal being taken as 100 per cent (see Prothrombin and Proconvertin Test).

PLASMA FIBRINOGEN

Fibrinogen is necessary for blood clotting, being converted by thrombin into fibrin which is the essential constituent of blood clot. For its estimation blood is collected in a Sequestrene or heparin bottle. Normally plasma fibrinogen is 2–4g/litre (200–400mg/100ml). This level increases during pregnancy. An abrupt fall in the fibrinogen to levels below 1g/litre (100mg/100ml) may occur in a pregnant woman when there is intra-uterine death of the fetus. This can lead to dangerous haemorrhage. A rapid method of estimating fibrinogen is therefore of great value. (See Fibrindex, below.) Low plasma fibrinogen also occurs in severe liver disease and as a congenital abnormality.

FIBRINDEX (Fibrinogen Index)

This test gives a quick estimate of the patient's fibrinogen level. 2ml of blood in a prothrombin bottle is required. The result is reported as the time taken for the patient's plasma to clot after it is added to thrombin. Normally it clots in 5–12 seconds. In moderate fibrinogen deficiency the time in 12–30 seconds. In severe deficiency it is over 30 seconds. It is chiefly used in obstetrical emergencies and following thoracic operations.

PROTHROMBIN CONSUMPTION TEST

When healthy blood clots most of the prothrombin is used up. In clotting defects much prothrombin may still remain in the serum. This test measures how much of the original plasma prothrombin remains in the serum. This is the pro-thrombin consumption index (PCI) normally 0–30 per cent, usually below 10 per cent. A raised result indicates a clotting defect requiring further investigation by one or more of the next three tests to be described.

THROMBOPLASTIN GENERATION TEST (Biggs and Douglas)

This test will detect deficiencies of certain blood clotting factors. In haemophilia it shows the antihaemophilic globulin to be deficient. In Christmas disease, the deficiency of the Christmas factor can be detected.

The test will also demonstrate the presence of circulating anticoagulants (pseudohaemophilia) and platelet defects. The blood is collected by the laboratory technician. A preliminary Thromboplastin Screening Test is usually performed, or alternatively the Kaolin Cephalin Time (see below).

KAOLIN CEPHALIN TIME

This is often used as an alternative to the Thromboplastin Screening Test in the preliminary investigation of a suspected coagulation defect. It is the time taken for plasma to clot when incubated in the presence of calcium, kaolin and cephalin (a platelet substitute made from brain). Normally the kaolin cephalin time is 45–60 seconds. It is prolonged in all coagulation defects except those due to defects or diminution of platelets or fibrinogen (laboratory collection).

FACTOR ASSAYS

In cases of haemorrhagic disorder it is now possible to identify exactly which factor(s) the patient lacks by means of factor assays.

FIBRINOLYSIN

Fibrinolysin is a substance causing lysis and breakdown of blood clot. If the clot remains solid after 24 hours' incubation the test is regarded as negative. Increased fibrinolysin is sometimes found after massive blood loss, after treatment with the heart-lung machine and occasionally in liver disease, heart failure and certain obstetric emergencies. Blood is collected by the laboratory technician.

STREPTOKINASE RESISTANCE TEST

Streptokinase is used in the treatment of thromboembolic disorders. It is obtained from purified filtrates of β-haemolytic streptococci. Streptokinase acts by converting inactive plasminogen into the protein-digesting enzyme plasmin. Plasmin digests fibrin and also other coagulation factors. The aim of treatment is to digest the fibrin without seriously affecting the other factors. This is achieved by using high doses of streptokinase which keeps the plasminogen at a low level. But patients who have had a recent streptococcal infection are liable to have antibodies. These have to be neutralised by a higher concentration of streptokinase, the dosage being determined by means of the streptokinase resistance test.

CAPILLARY MICROSCOPY

The capillaries at the base of the fingernails may be examined under the microscope, using an Angle-poise lamp and a drop of immersion oil on the nail bed. Vascular abnormality such as increased capillary tortuosity may be demonstrated, usually associated with a prolonged bleeding time.

Investigations for the Haemolytic Anaemias
(i.e. anaemias due to destruction of circulating red cells)

HAEMOGLOBIN ESTIMATION (see p. 45)

An unexplained fall in the haemoglobin level may be the presenting feature of a haemolytic anaemia.

BLOOD FILM (see p. 49, Red Cell Appearance)

Certain features may suggest a haemolytic anaemia, e.g. small densely-staining red cells (apparent microspherocytes); considerable polychromasia or reticulocytosis (see p. 49); nucleated red cells ('normoblastic showers'); elliptical red cells (elliptocytes); red cell fragments; also target cells, poikilocytes and iron deficiency changes.

HAPTOGLOBIN

Haptoglobin is a serum protein, a globulin with a large molecule. The normal range is 0.3–2.0g/litre (30–200mg/100ml). The level is reduced in haemolytic anaemia. This provides a convenient method for detecting a haemolytic condition. It is estimated either chemically or by electrophoresis, 10ml of clotted blood being required. The haptoglobin level is also reduced in glandular fever, liver diseases and the rare congenital deficiency of hapto-globin (ahaptoglobinaemia). The haptoglobin level is increased in infections, malignancy including Hodgkin's disease, tissue damage, systemic lupus erythematosus and in steroid therapy.

WET FILM

A drop of blood diluted with normal saline is examined microscopically. Small spherical red cells (microsphero-cytes) or elliptical red cells (elliptocytes) may be seen.

TESTS FOR SICKLING AND HAEMOGLOBIN S

The amount of oxygen in a drop of diluted blood is lowered artificially. This produces sickle-shaped (crescent-shaped) cells in sickle cell anaemia, the most severe of the haemoly-tic anaemias. It is an hereditary condition, characteristically affecting negroes of African origin, due to the presence of abnormal haemoglobin S in the red cells. Recently developed tests are based on the fact that haemoglobin S is converted into crystals by reducing agents.

DIRECT COOMBS' TEST (see p. 69)

BLOOD GROUP

Haemolytic disease of the newborn results from a difference in blood group between mother and fetus, usually of the Rhesus type, as described on p. 64.

SERUM BILIRUBIN (see pp. 20, 22)

This is only raised if there is much haemolysis.

RED CELL OSMOTIC FRAGILITY

Red blood cells are stable in normal saline because its osmotic pressure is equal to that inside the cells. If the osmotic pressure is reduced by diluting the saline, a point is reached when the cells burst. This is known as haemolysis.

In certain haemolytic anaemias, e.g. acholuric jaundice and the acquired haemolytic anaemias, the red cells are more fragile, and haemolysis occurs with less dilute solutions of saline than normally. 10ml of heparinised blood is required for the fragility test.

The result, usually accompanied by a graph, is given thus:
Normal control—
    Haemolysis commences at 0.45 per cent.
    Haemolysis is complete at 0.35 per cent.
Acholuric jaundice—
    Haemolysis commences at 0.6 per cent.
    Haemolysis is complete at 0.45 per cent.
In certain haemolytic anaemias the red cells are more resistant than normal against low osmotic pressures, e.g. Mediterranean anaemia and sickle cell anaemia.

ANTIBODIES (see p. 66)

In haemolytic anaemia with a positive direct Coombs' test, e.g. the acquired haemolytic anaemias, antibody can be obtained (eluted) from the surface of the patient's red cells and then tested against various known red cells.

HAEMOLYSINS

These are antibodies which cause the red cells to rupture. They are demonstrated by incubating the patient's serum with suitable suspensions of red cells under certain conditions, viz warmth, cold and acidity. An example is Ham's Test for a haemolysin active in acidified serum: it is positive in paroxysmal nocturnal haemoglobinuria. Fresh specimens are essential, preferably collected by the laboratory staff. Sometimes two specimens are required, one being placed immediately in a water bath at 37°C to clot and the other in an ice bath at 0°C. This is necessary to detect the cold antibody causing paroxysmal cold haemoglobinuria by the Donath-Landsteiner Test.

AUTOHAEMOLYSIS

This test is performed to help diagnose hereditary spherocytosis and to a lesser extent other types of haemolytic anaemia. From a fresh sample of clotted blood the red cells are incubated at 37°C in their own serum with and without added glucose. Normal values after 48 hours incubation are:

> Without added glucose, 0.2–2 per cent haemolysis
> With added glucose, 0.01–0.9 per cent

Haemolytic red cells show increased haemolysis without added glucose, which is corrected to some degree by added glucose.

ABNORMAL HAEMOGLOBINS

Some forms of haemolytic anaemia are due to the red cells containing abnormal haemoglobin as a congenital anomaly. Mediterranean anaemia (thalassaemia) is a typical example, in which a certain proportion of the haemoglobin is of the type normally found in the fetus, known as fetal haemoglobin. This may be detected by the alkali resistance test, fetal haemoglobin being abnormally resistant to alkali. 10ml of heparinised blood is sufficient for both this and the following tests.

Other types of haemoglobin, such as that found in sickle

cell anaemia and similar congenital abnormalities, may be detected by electrophoresis. Sufficient for this test may be obtained by finger-prick. (See also Tests for Sickling and Haemoglobin S, p. 59.)

Abnormal haemoglobin may also result from certain drugs and poisons such as chlorates and carbon monoxide, also following incompatible blood transfusion. These may be detected by spectroscopy. For this test about 2ml of sequestrenated, heparinised or oxalated blood should be sent to the laboratory.

GLUCOSE 6 PHOSPHATE DEHYDROGENASE (G 6 PD) DEFICIENCY

Some people are born with red cells lacking an enzyme called glucose 6 phosphate dehydrogenase. This inherited defect only becomes evident on exposure to certain drugs or chemicals such as the sulphones of naphthalene (moth-balls) which cause the red cells to break down, resulting in haemolytic anaemia. The haemolytic process stops when exposure to the offending substance ceases. The following tests are of value:

1. Heinz Body Test
Incubation of the defective cells with a reducing agent, e.g. acetyl phenylhydrazine, causes more Heinz bodies to develop than in normal blood.

2. Glutathione Stability Test
Defective cells incubated as above contain less reduced glutathione than normal cells.

3. Methaemoglobin Reduction Test
Defective cells accelerate the reduction of methaemo-globin under appropriate conditions.

4. Assay of Glucose 6 Phosphate Dehydrogenase Activity
This is the most reliable test and is now available in many laboratories.

Blood for the above tests is collected by the laboratory staff.

RED CELL SURVIVAL

The shortened length of life of the red cells in haemolytic anaemias can be demonstrated in two ways:

1. Ashby's method
Blood of a compatible but slightly different blood group is transfused into the patient. Samples of blood are then collected, daily for the first week and then at longer intervals, usually by finger-prick. The transfused cells can be recognised by their blood group, and their time of survival measured.

2. Radio-isotope method
Red cells, preferably from the patient himself, are tagged with radioactive chromium and re-injected into the patient's bloodstream. By measuring the radioactivity with an instrument like a Geiger counter the life span of the red cells can be estimated.

SCHUMM'S TEST

When haemolysis occurs in the bloodstream, e.g. following incompatible blood transfusion and in certain haemolytic anaemias, methaemalbumin is released from the haemolysed cells. This is detected in the plasma or serum by Schumm's test, using spectroscopy. (See also p. 69.)

URINE TESTS

Urobilin (see p. 19) is increased in haemolytic anaemias, especially during an active phase. Haemoglobin appears in the urine in certain severe haemolytic anaemias, e.g. paroxysmal nocturnal haemoglobinuria.

Blood Groups

There are four main blood groups:

A   B   AB   O

Of the population of the United Kingdom:

47 per cent are group O

42 per cent are group A

8 per cent are group B

3 per cent are group AB

Russians, Arabs, and Turks show a higher percentage of group B.

To ascertain a person's blood group, his cells are placed against known sera; thus A cells are agglutinated by anti-A serum, but not by anti-B serum.

B cells are agglutinated by anti-B serum and not by anti-A serum. AB cells are agglutinated by both sera and O cells are not agglutinated by either.

A person's blood group is named after the antigens in his red cells. In practice it is checked by also testing for the antibodies in his serum. Thus group A blood contains anti-B antibody in the serum; group B blood contains anti-A antibody; group O blood contains both antibodies; and group AB blood contains neither.

It is the presence of these antibodies that makes it vital that blood of the right group is selected for blood transfusion. In addition to ABO there are other blood group systems, the most important being the Rhesus (Rh) type described below. Less commonly investigated blood groups include MNS, P, Kell, Duffy, Kidd, Lewis, etc. More are being discovered.

The fact that blood groups are inherited is of legal importance in cases of disputed paternity of a child.

RHESUS TYPE

Eighty-five per cent of the population are Rhesus positive. This means that their cells are agglutinated by a serum which also agglutinates the cells of a rhesus monkey. People whose cells are not agglutinated by the serum are Rhesus negative.

This is of importance in haemolytic disease of the newborn as well as in blood transfusion.

A Rhesus negative mother and a Rhesus positive father may have a Rhesus positive child, and in a small percentage of cases the mother produces antibodies which pass through the placenta and damage the red cells of the fetus. As a result, the baby may be stillborn, or else develop severe jaundice and anaemia shortly after birth. This condition does not occur in the first pregnancy, unless the mother has previously been stimulated to produce antibodies—e.g. by transfusion with Rhesus positive blood.

Haemolytic disease of the newborn may also be due to other types of incompatibility, in the Rhesus, ABO or other blood group systems.

ANTENATAL BLOOD TESTS

All pregnant women should have an antenatal blood test during the third or fourth month. A venepuncture sample is taken into three containers—2ml sequestrenated blood for haemoglobin estimation, 5ml clotted blood for rubella and syphilis antibodies (see pp. 74–6, 78), and 5ml clotted blood for grouping. The latter is Rhesus typed and the serum screened for antibodies (see Antibody Testing, p. 66). All Rhesus negative women are ABO grouped and if they have no living children they are booked for hospital delivery (see Kleihauer Test, p. 66). If an antibody is detected it is identified and the husband's blood group investigated (genotyped) to assess the probable outcome in this and future pregnancies. Women with antibodies have a blood sample taken each month for the antibody level (titre) to be measured. If a sharp rise in titre is found, measures may be instituted to monitor and protect the baby, e.g. amniocentesis (see p. 162), early induction of labour, exchange transfusion of baby, or in severe cases intra-uterine transfusion.

KLEIHAUER TEST FOR FETAL CELLS IN MATERNAL BLOOD

This test is of value in the prevention of haemolytic disease of the newborn. A sequestrenated sample of blood is collected from the mother at exactly 10 minutes after delivery. When treated with acid and the stained film examined microscopically the fetal cells stand out quite clearly and can be counted. If fetal cells are detected in the mother's blood and the baby is Rhesus positive with the same ABO group as the mother, she is in danger of being stimulated to produce Rhesus antibody. This can be prevented by injecting the mother with Rhesus Antibody within 36 hours of delivery, destroying the fetal cells before they have time to sensitise her. This procedure is being adopted for all Rhesus negative women.

ROUTINE TESTS FOR HAEMOLYTIC DISEASE OF THE NEWBORN

As soon as a baby with suspected haemolytic disease is born the following samples should be sent to the laboratory:
(a) from the mother—two 5ml samples of clotted blood; one 2ml sample of sequestrenated blood.
(b) from the baby (cord blood)—10ml of clotted blood; 5ml of clotted blood; 2ml of sequestrenated blood.

A positive direct Coombs' test (p. 69) indicates that the baby has haemolytic disease; its nature is revealed by the blood groups. The baby's haemoglobin and serum bilirubin levels give guidance on the severity of the condition and indicate whether exchange transfusion is required.

Antibody Testing

The patient's serum is tested against cells having known antigens, including the patient's own cells. By finding which antigen is common to all the cells which are agglutinated by the serum, the antibody can be named. More than one antibody may be present. (See also Antenatal Blood Tests, p. 65.)

BLOOD TRANSFUSION

The chief importance of blood groups is in blood transfusion. For example, if group A blood is transfused into a patient who is group O, the transfused cells will be agglutinated and haemolysed by the antibodies present in the patient. The patient will suffer a severe reaction, with jaundice and kidney failure, which may result in death. It is therefore essential that blood used for transfusion is compatible with the patient's blood, wherever possible of the same group and Rhesus type. All patients likely to require blood transfusion should therefore be grouped and Rhesus typed at the earliest opportunity. Where transfusion is certain, the blood must also be cross-matched. This entails placing the red cells of the donor with serum of the patient and then examining for agglutination. Grouping and cross-matching normally takes a minimum of four hours. For this purpose, about 5ml of blood are collected in a dry sterile tube and sent to the laboratory. It must be fully labelled with forenames, surname, age, address and ward and accompanied by a fully completed request form. If there is a history of previous transfusions, or if the patient is a woman whose children have had haemolytic disease at birth or gives a history of miscarriage, these facts must be stated on the request form.

The Regional Blood Transfusion Centres play an important part by collecting the blood from the donors, grouping it and distributing it to all hospitals.

To help to identify the different blood groups an International colour code is used for the bottle labels:

Yellow for A
Pink   for B

White   for AB
Blue   for O

Rhesus negative blood has red lettering and a red vertical stripe. Rhesus positive blood has black lettering with no vertical stripe.

It is vital that the bottles of blood are stored in a refrigerator with a rigidly controlled temperature of 4°C and an alarm system to warn if temperature varies. Blood must not be stored in an ordinary ward or domestic refrigerator (unless specially modified) and must not be warmed or frozen. It may be kept for up to 3 hours in an insulated transporting box freshly issued from the blood bank.

THE INVESTIGATION OF TRANSFUSION REACTIONS

Transfusion reactions may be either non-haemolytic or haemolytic.

a. *Non-haemolytic reactions* include pyrexial and allergic reactions to the transfusion fluid, circulatory overloading, air embolism (more likely if positive pressure is used) and septicaemia from infected transfusion fluid. The latter can be proved only by isolating the same organism from the patient and from the transfusion fluid. This is one reason for not destroying or washing out the bottles or packs after transfusion.

b. *Haemolytic reactions* result from the destruction of either donor or recipient red cells following transfusion. The following must be available for investigation:

1. The remains of all transfused fluids (blood, plasma, saline, etc).
2. Two post-transfusion samples of blood from the recipient: 10ml of clotted blood, 10ml of citrated blood, collected from a vein well away from the transfusion site.
3. All urine passed after the transfusion reaction.

4. A pre-transfusion blood sample should be available in the blood bank.

Typical findings following a haemolytic transfusion reaction are as follows:

	Pre-transfusion	Post-transfusion
Serum Bilirubin	Normal	Raised
Serum Haptoglobin	Normal	Reduced
Direct Coombs' Test	Negative	Positive
Schumm's Test (p. 63)	Negative	Positive
Free Haemoglobin in Plasma	Absent	Present

COOMBS' TEST

The presence of antibodies coating the red cells, e.g. of a newborn baby with haemolytic disease, may be detected by Coombs' reagent which causes the cells to agglutinate. Coombs' reagent is also known as anti-human globulin since it contains antibodies active against human globulins. Rhesus antibody and all other antibodies are globulin. Coombs' reagent will thus detect the presence of any antibody coating the red cell.

Coated red cells which agglutinate with Coombs' reagent are said to give a positive Coombs' test. If washed cells direct from the patient are found to be so agglutinated it is reported as a positive Direct Coombs' test. In addition to haemolytic disease of the newborn, a positive Direct Coombs' test may be found in acquired haemolytic anaemia. This indicates that the patient has produced antibodies against his own red cells (an example of auto-immunity). Following mis-matched blood transfusion, blood from the patient gives a positive direct Coombs' test, the donor cells being coated with antibody from the patient.

Coombs' reagent may also be used to detect antibodies in the serum. After appropriate cells have been placed in contact with the serum they are washed and then tested for antibody coating, using Coombs' reagent. This is known as the Indirect Coombs' test. It forms the basis of the Coombs' cross-match, donor's cells being incubated in patient's serum, washed, and then tested for coating.

GAMMA GLOBULIN NEUTRALISATION TEST

This distinguishes between antibody of gamma globulin type and that of non-gamma globulin type. Gamma globulin antibody is likely to be of importance in causing haemolytic disease of the newborn. Non-gamma globulin is unlikely to. About 5ml of clotted blood is required. Coombs' reagent neutralised with gamma globulin no longer reacts with cells coated by antibody which is gamma globulin. It continues to react with cells coated by antibody which is non-gamma globulin.

Other Tests in Haematology

TESTS FOR GLANDULAR FEVER

1. Paul-Bunnell Test
This test is positive in many cases of glandular fever. The patient's serum is found to agglutinate the red cells from a sheep, even after considerable dilution of the serum. A finger-prick sample is sufficient for a preliminary screening test. If this is positive a full test must be done, requiring 5ml of clotted blood.

2. Monospot and Monosticon
These are proprietary tests for glandular fever similar in principle to the Paul-Bunnell but more rapid. A positive Monospot or Monosticon with a positive Paul-Bunnell screening test may be considered diagnostic of glandular fever.

TESTS FOR RHEUMATOID ARTHRITIS

1. Differential Agglutination Test (DAT, Rose's test, Rose-Waaler test). Also called Sheep Cell Agglutination Test (SCAT)

Serum from many patients with rheumatoid arthritis agglutinates sheep red cells which have been specially sensitised. A DAT of 1 in 16 or more is regarded as positive. Positive results are found most frequently in adult rheumatoid arthritis and in systemic lupus erythematosus, less frequently in childhood rheumatoid arthritis (Still's disease) and in hepatitis. 5–10ml of clotted blood is required.

2. Hyland RA Test

A drop of diluted patient's serum is tested on a slide against latex particles coated with γ-globulin. Agglutination of the particles is reported as a positive test. The results usually correspond to those with the DAT.

It is best to use both tests in each case, the results being most reliable when the two tests agree.

TESTS FOR DISSEMINATED (SYSTEMIC) LUPUS ERYTHEMATOSUS

1. LE (Lupus Erythematosus) 'Cell Preparation' Test

5–10ml of fresh clotted blood is required. In the laboratory it is appropriately incubated and smears of the white cells examined. Cells, usually polymorphs, containing large round masses of structureless material are reported as LE cells. Their finding strongly suggests systematic lupus erythematosus.

2. Hyland LE Test

A drop of the patient's serum is tested on a slide against latex particles coated with nucleoprotein. Agglutination of the particles is reported as a positive test. The results usually correspond to the 'cell preparation' test and are most reliable when the two tests agree.

3. Anti-nuclear Factor (ANF)

Serum from patients with systemic lupus erythematosus may contain a factor which reacts with the nuclei of normal human cells. This can be demonstrated on a slide using the fluorescent antibody technique (see below). A positive result strongly supports the diagnosis of systemic lupus erythematosus.

FLUORESCENT ANTIBODY TECHNIQUE

This technique can be used to detect the presence of anti-body in the patient's blood against various tissue elements, e.g. thyroid in auto-immune thyroid disease (p. 187), stomach in pernicious anaemia, or nuclei of any tissue in DLE (see Anti-nuclear Factor above).

The patient's serum is layered over a section or smear of fresh tissue. Any antibody present will then combine with the corresponding tissue element. All the uncombined serum is washed off. Antibody being a globulin can be demonstrated by adding a fluorescent anti-globulin and examining microscopically.

BACTERICIDAL ACTIVITY (NitroBlue Tetrazolium, NBT)

For this test 20ml of venous blood is collected into a mix-ture of heparin and dextran. The dextran causes the red cells to form rouleaux and sediment rapidly, leaving the leucocytes in suspension. After treatment with tetrazolium, the actively bactericidal cells show a deep blue precipitate when examined under the microscope. During infections more than 50 per cent of the cells show this change in normal people. In patients with granulomatous disease less than 10 per cent of the cells show evidence of bactericidal activity.

Part II. Bacteriological Tests on Blood

BLOOD CULTURES

The circulating blood is normally sterile and any isolated organisms gaining entrance to the circulation are rapidly destroyed by the body's defences. In septicaemia, living organisms are present in considerable numbers in the bloodstream. The presence of septicaemia may be suspected in cases of septic illness with recurrent high temperature and rigors. Its presence may be confirmed by blood culture.

For this purpose about 10ml of blood are taken from a vein after the skin has been disinfected with 70% alcohol, e.g. Medi-Swab. The blood is transferred aseptically into bottles containing suitable broth culture media. These are then placed in an incubator for up to a fortnight or longer.

Repeated cultures may have to be done to obtain a positive result in cases of septicaemia.

Blood cultures are especially useful in the diagnosis of puerperal sepsis, endocarditis, typhoid fever in the early stages, and all cases of pyrexia of undetermined origin. Cultures of blood should be taken before antibacterial drugs are administered.

WIDAL REACTION FOR TYPHOID, PARATYPHOID AND BRUCELLOSIS (Abortus and Undulant fevers)

A person with any of the above infections usually develops corresponding antibodies 7–10 days after the onset of the disease. The antibodies are called agglutinins because of their ability to agglutinate or clump suspensions of bacteria causing the infection. The strength of the antibody increases during the disease. This is demonstrated by the increasing dilution (rising titre) of the patient's serum at which the antibody can be detected.

In people who have been vaccinated with TAB (killed organisms of typhoid, paratyphoid A and B) in the past some antibody will be found in the serum, but a rising titre on repeat test is strong evidence of active infection.

In a suspected case of any of these diseases 5ml of clotted blood are collected in a dry tube and sent to the laboratory, where the serum is tested as described.

The Vi test. This is a special type of agglutination test, used mainly to demonstrate the typhoid carrier state.

Additional serological tests (Coombs' and complement fixation tests) are useful in the diagnosis of brucellosis.

Blood Tests for Syphilis

The blood tests most commonly used for screening for syphilitic infection are the Venereal Disease Reference Laboratory (VDRL) slide test and the Treponema Pallidum HaemAgglutination (TPHA) test. The Wassermann Reaction (WR) and the Reiter Protein Complement Fixation Test (RPCFT) are now being replaced by the above tests. 5ml of clotted blood is sufficient for the tests. If an equivocal or unexpected result is obtained the tests are repeated, and then if necessary blood may be referred to the VD reference laboratory. The essence of all the tests is the demonstration of the syphilitic antibody.

VENEREAL DISEASE REFERENCE LABORATORY
(VDRL) SLIDE TEST

This test usually becomes positive 7–10 days after the appearance of the chancre. It is a satisfactory and rapid screening test. It has taken the place of the Wassermann Reaction for monitoring treatment. Like the WR, it can give a false biological positive reaction.

TREPONEMA PALLIDUM HAEMAGGLUTINATION
(TPHA) TEST

This is a sensitive test for antibody in all stages of syphilis. It cannot be used for monitoring treatment because it remains positive for a very long time, even after cure. In this respect it resembles the Treponema Immobilisation Test (TIT or TPI) and the Fluorescent Treponemal Antibody Test (FTAT).

The TPHA test rarely gives rise to a false biological positive reaction. The FTAT only very rarely gives such a reaction.

WASSERMANN REACTION (WR)

This usually becomes positive 6 to 8 weeks after infection. Successful treatment early in the disease usually causes it to become negative fairly quickly. Long-standing cases may never become negative. The test may also be done on cerebrospinal fluid.

The results may be classified as positive (+), doubtful (±) or negative (−). Sometimes the result may be given according to the titre, i.e. dilution of serum at which antibody can just be detected. With much antibody the titre is high, e.g. 1 in 40. With less antibody the titre is lower, e.g. 1 in 5.

The test may give a positive reaction temporarily during the course of various diseases or pregnancy in persons who have not had syphilis.

REITER PROTEIN COMPLEMENT FIXATION TEST (Reiter Protein CFT or RPCFT)

This test is being replaced by the VDRL and TPHA tests (p. 74) as screening tests. The antigen used is from a strain of Treponema pallidum, the organism which causes syphilis, and so in theory this is a more specific test than the others. In practice the use of the above two screening tests is found to detect more cases of syphilis than any one test alone.

CONFIRMATORY TESTS FOR SYPHILIS

The most important are the Treponema Immobilisation Test (TIT or TPI), the VDRL Flocculation Test and the Fluorescent Treponemal Antibody Test (FTAT).

Blood Test for Gonorrhoea

Gonococcal Fixation Test (GCFT). This is a test for the gonococcal antibody. 2–5ml of clotted blood are required. It is only of value where chronic gonococcal infection is suspected, e.g. with joint complications.

Blood Tests for Antibodies to Other Infections

ASPERGILLOSIS (about 5ml of clotted blood is required)

The demonstration of serum antibodies to the fungus Aspergillus fumigatus assists in the diagnosis. The patient's serum and antigens from A. fumigatus are allowed to diffuse towards each other in agar gel ('agar gel diffusion'). A line of precipitation where the two meet indicates the presence of antibody to A. fumigatus. A positive result is of great value in interpreting the finding of fungus in the sputum, indicating infection and not just contamination.

AUSTRALIA (HEPATITIS B) ANTIGEN (5ml of clotted blood is required)

The presence of Australia antigen in the blood is associated with serum hepatitis which is now an industrial disease.

CANDIDA ALBICANS (5ml of clotted blood is required)

The diagnosis of systemic Candida albicans infection by the demonstration of antibodies in the patient's serum has recently been developed. The method used is agar gel diffusion as for aspergillosis (see above), using instead antigens from Candida albicans.

COCCIDIOIDOMYCOSIS (5ml of clotted blood is required)

The demonstration of serum antibodies to the fungus C. immitis assists diagnosis. See also Coccidioidin skin test (p. 234).

FARMER'S LUNG (5ml of clotted blood is required)

This is an allergic condition due to inhalation of dust from mouldy hay. Antibodies to hay moulds are present in about 90 per cent of patients with farmer's lung. These can be detected by either agar gel diffusion or immuno-electrophoresis.

HISTOPLASMOSIS (5ml of clotted blood is required)

The demonstration of serum antibodies to the fungus Histoplasma capsulatum assists in the diagnosis of this infection. See also Histoplasmin skin test (p. 235).

HYDATID DISEASE (5ml of clotted blood is required)

Immunological diagnosis of hydatid disease can be made by the demonstration of antibodies in the patient's serum.

LEGIONNAIRE'S DISEASE (5ml clotted blood required)

Antibodies to the causative organism, Legionella pneumophila, may not be demonstrable until 3–4 weeks after infection. During the acute phase the organism can be cultured from sputum but at present only a few laboratories have the necessary facilities.

LEPTOSPIRA ANTIBODIES (10ml of clotted blood is required)

The patient's serum may be tested in three ways:

1. Agglutination and lysis of live leptospira.
2. Agglutination of dead formalised leptospira.
3. Complement fixation test.

The tests become positive at about the tenth day in Weil's disease (due to Leptospira icterohaemorrhagiae) and in infection by the dog leptospira (L. canicola).

RUBELLA (GERMAN MEASLES) ANTIBODIES (5ml of clotted blood is required)

Rubella infection in the first three months of pregnancy can cause congenital abnormalities, e.g. heart disease in the fetus. So it is now becoming routine practice for blood to be sent for rubella antibody (and syphilis serology) testing at the first antenatal attendance. An antibody titre of 1 in 32 is consistent with immunity from previous infection. Less than 1 in 32 indicates lack of immunity and the mother is warned of the danger to the fetus of exposure to rubella. A titre of over 1 in 64 suggests possible infection and a repeat should be undertaken. A rising titre, associated with a high IgM level, indicates active infection. Rubella during the first three months of pregnancy is now considered to warrant therapeutic abortion.

STREPTOCOCCAL ASO (ANTI-STREPTOLYSIN 'O') TITRE (5ml of clotted blood is required)

Patients infected with haemolytic streptococcus develop antibodies, particularly against the 'O' haemolysin, reaching their maximum 2 to 4 weeks after infection. An ASO titre of 200 or above implies recent streptococcal infection. Under the age of 5 years a lower titre may be significant. It is of value in determining the cause of rheumatic fever, erythema nodosum, nephritis and allied conditions.

SCHISTOSOMIASIS (5ml of clotted blood is required)

Demonstration of serum antibodies to schistosomes is of value in the diagnosis of chronic infections when microscopy of urine, faeces and tissue has proved negative.

STAPHYLOCOCCAL ANTIBODIES (5ml of clotted blood is required)

Two antibody tests, anti-α-haemolysin and anti-leucocidin, especially the former, are of value in ascertaining whether hidden staphylococcal infection is present, e.g. osteomyelitis.

TOXOPLASMA ANTIBODIES (5ml of clotted blood is required)

Toxoplasma antibodies are usually detected by means of a dye test. The demonstration of an antibody indicates infection with toxoplasma, either present or past. Active infection may be inferred either from a high antibody titre of over 1/256 or from a rising titre when the test is repeated after an interval of 2 weeks. About a third of normal adults have a titre of 1/8 to 1/128, indicating past infection.

ANTIBODIES IN PRIMARY ATYPICAL PNEUMONIA

Most patients with primary atypical pneumonia develop antibodies which can be detected by a complement fixation test. Two samples of about 5ml of clotted blood are required, one early in the disease and one late or during convalescence. A rising titre is diagnostic.

ANTIBODY TESTS IN OTHER INFECTIOUS DISEASES

Two 10ml samples of clotted blood, one taken as early as possible during the disease and the second about a fortnight later, provide similar diagnostic information in many infectious diseases including virus infections (see p. 232) and many parasitic infestations, e.g. trypanosomiasis, leishmaniasis, cysticercosis, fascioliasis (liver fluke), filariasis, leishmaniasis (including kala-azar) and trichiniasis (see also p. 236).

Part III. Chemical Tests on Blood

ALCOHOL

This test is being carried out with increasing frequency in police cases to ascertain whether a person is under the influence of alcohol in connection with various offences, e.g. motor accidents, etc.

About 5ml of blood are sent to the laboratory in a plain tube. Some other bodies in the blood, e.g. acetone, are estimated as alcohol, and for this reason a normal estimation may be up to 0.4g/litre (40mg/100ml) of blood.

Blood levels in alcoholic intoxication:

slight	0.8–1.0g/litre	(80–100mg/100ml)
obvious	1.5g/litre	(150mg/100ml)
stupor	3.0g/litre	(300mg/100ml)

(urine levels are usually slightly higher)

ALDOSTERONE

See under adrenal gland investigations, p. 191.

ALKALI RESISTANCE (ALKALI DENATURATION) TEST

See abnormal haemoglobin, p. 61.

ALPHA$_1$ (α_1) ANTITRYPSIN

This is a glycoprotein involved in the response to acute infections and tissue damage. These conditions cause a raised serum level unless there is a congenital deficiency of α_1 antitrypsin. Deficiency is associated with neonatal cholestasis, juvenile cirrhosis and emphysema, with a lowered resistance to lung infections and a great susceptibility to the effects of smoking. About 5ml of clotted blood are required for the test. It must be collected *without a tourniquet* and sent immediately to the laboratory. The request form should summarise the results of liver or lung function

tests, liver biopsy or chest x-ray findings, family history of
lung disease and urine findings. Family studies on close
relatives of an affected individual provide a basis for
genetic counselling.

ALPHAFETO-PROTEIN (AFP)

This is a glycoprotein produced by the liver of the fetus and
greatly reduced after birth. The normal adult serum level is
$2-25\mu g$/litre. During pregnancy the maternal serum level
is usually below $100\mu g$/litre between the 14th–18th weeks;
it reaches its maximum of $30-500\mu g$/litre between the
28th–36th weeks. In the newborn it is $50-150\mu g$/litre,
decreasing to the normal adult level by 5 weeks. In view of
the wide range, units must be carefully checked (viz ng, μg,
g/ml, litre).

Estimation is of value in (1) tumour diagnosis and
monitoring, (2) detection of the fetal abnormalities and (3)
other conditions.

(1) Serum AFP is raised in most (80–90 per cent)
hepatocellular carcinomas and hepatoblastomas, many
malignant teratomas, some alimentary tract carcinomas
and secondary tumours of liver and occasionally other
tumours. Estimation before surgery (e.g. gonadectomy)
and about 2 weeks afterwards provides a guide to com-
pleteness of removal. It can also be used to monitor
radiotherapy.

(2) The pregnancy serum level is raised in anencephaly,
spinal tubal defects and fetal death (see also *Amniocentesis*, p. 162).

(3) Raised serum AFP occurs in hepatitis, especially in
children. It is said to indicate a favourable prognosis in any
acute liver failure. It is also raised in cirrhosis, biliary atresia
and ataxia telangiectasia.

No preparation of the patient is required. About 5ml
clotted blood should be sent to the laboratory early in the
day.

AMINO-ACIDS

1. Total amino-acid nitrogen. 10ml of heparinised blood are required. Normal blood contains less than 80mg/litre (8mg/100ml) amino-acid nitrogen. Increased levels occur in liver and kidney failure.
2. Phenylalanine, see p. 96.

ASCORBIC ACID (VITAMIN C)

5ml of anticoagulated blood are required. Normally 10–100μmol/litre (0.4–2.0mg/100ml) are present. Below 10μmol/litre (0.2mg/100ml) suggests scurvy. The saturation test (see p. 252) is more reliable than a blood estimation.

BILIRUBIN (see pp. 19–22)

BROMSULPHALEIN (see Intravenous Dye Test, p. 22)

CALCIUM AND MAGNESIUM

Some 5ml of blood are collected *without a tourniquet* into a dry tube and sent to the laboratory. The normal **calcium** is 2.1–2.6mmol/litre (8.5–10.5mg/100ml), slightly higher in young children. (Since half the calcium is bound to albumin the above values depend on a normal albumin level.) Symptoms of tetany occur when the figure is as low as 1.5mmol/litre (6mg/100ml). Low readings are found in tetany, renal dwarfism, osteomalacia, coeliac disease, in some cases of rickets and in chronic nephritis. High readings may be found in cases of parathyroid tumour (causing generalised osteitis fibrosa) sarcoidosis and vitamin D excess.

Serum **magnesium**, normally 0.6–1mmol/litre (1.5–2.6mg/100ml), may be estimated on the same specimen. Low levels may occur in tetany and renal failure.

INORGANIC PHOSPHATE (PHOSPHORUS)

5ml of blood are collected into a plain dry container and sent to the laboratory without delay. The normal phosphate is 0.8–1.45mmol/litre (2.5–4.5mg P/100ml) for adults and 1.3–1.9mmol/litre for children. It is raised in chronic nephritis, prolonged diabetic coma, hyperparathyroidism, rickets and osteomalacia.

ALKALINE PHOSPHATASE

About 5ml of blood are sent to the laboratory in a dry tube. The normal figure is 10–40iu/litre (3–13 King Armstrong units/100ml) in adults and 20–70iu/litre in children and during pregnancy. It is raised in cirrhosis of the liver, obstructive jaundice and many bone diseases including rickets and hyperparathyroidism. To determine whether a raised serum alkaline phosphatase is of liver or bone origin 5-nucleotidase estimation may be undertaken (p. 94).

Note. Calcium, phosphorus and alkaline phosphatase are frequently estimated on the same specimen. A single 5ml sample of clotted blood suffices.

ACID PHOSPHATASE

About 5ml of blood are sent to the laboratory in a dry tube. The normal figure is 2–7iu/litre (1–4 King Armstrong units/100ml). In carcinoma of the prostate it rises, especially when secondary growths are present.

CALCITONIN

This hormone, produced by the thyroid, inhibits the resorption of calcium from bone. The normal serum level is 20–400pg/ml. It is raised in medullary carcinoma of thyroid, also in pseudohypoparathyroidism, some renal disease and occasionally in breast, lung and other malignancies. A reduced level, occurring in hypoparathyroidism, is not demonstrable by routine assay. The laboratory should be contacted before collecting 10ml blood into an ice-cooled heparin tube.

CARBOXYHAEMOGLOBIN

This is found in poisoning from a car exhaust, products of combustion from oil heaters, fires and smouldering material and from coal gas; all contain carbon monoxide. (See p. 62.)

CARCINO-EMBRYONIC ANTIGEN (CEA)

This antigen was first demonstrated in carcinoma of the colon and in embryonic intestine. It is not specific for malignancy but may be used to monitor the course of some tumours. The normal serum level is less than $3\mu g$/litre, $3–10\mu g$/litre being borderline. It is raised in many conditions including heavy smoking (more than 15/day), chronic lung disease, peptic ulcer, inflammatory bowel disease and cirrhosis. Values above $20\mu g$/litre are suggestive of malignancy and above $50\mu g$/litre highly suggestive. In advanced malignancy the level may fall. About 5ml clotted blood should be sent to the laboratory early in the day.

CHOLESTEROL

10ml of blood are collected in a heparinised tube. The estimation is done on plasma in which the normal level is 3.6–5.7mmol/litre (140–220mg/100ml) at 20 years of age. It increases gradually with age.

The figure is raised in long continued biliary obstruction and in some cases of chronic nephritis (with proteinuria), diabetes, myxoedema and pregnancy.

The figure may be decreased in thyrotoxicosis, liver disease and chronic wasting diseases.

COMPLEMENT COMPONENTS C_3 AND C_4

The term 'complement' includes a number of enzymes in blood involved in immunity and activated by antigen-antibody complexes. Serum C_3 and C_4 levels are generally a guide to overall complement activity; the normal range for C_3 is 0.7–1.6g/litre and for C_4 is 0.1–0.5g/litre. They are raised in many conditions involving inflammation, e.g. infections, injuries and infarction. Reduced levels are of more diagnostic value and occur in acute nephritis, chronic membrano-proliferative nephritis and disseminated lupus erythematosus (DLE). About 5ml of freshly taken clotted blood is required.

(COMPLEMENT) C_1 ESTERASE INHIBITOR

This is a globulin which inhibits activated complement, limiting its possibly harmful effects. It is deficient in sufferers from Hereditary AngioNeurotic (o)Edema (HANE) who develop episodic swelling of various parts of the body, sometimes with serious effects. If detected, family studies are indicated. In the active phase C_4 is also low but C_3 is usually normal (see preceding section). About 5ml of freshly collected blood is required.

CONGO RED TEST

This test is of value in the diagnosis of amyloidosis.

The dye is injected intravenously, and samples of blood are collected after 4 and 60 minutes. From this the percentage of the dye absorbed from the blood in 1 hour can be calculated. Normally this is less than 50 per cent. In amyloidosis 90 per cent or more may be absorbed in 1 hour. A specimen of urine should also be collected at the end of the test, the bladder being empty at the commencement.

A false positive may be found in nephrosis. This is detected by the presence of a large part of the dye in the urine.

COPPER AND CAERULOPLASMIN

The normal serum copper is 13–25µmol/litre (70–150µg/100ml). Caeruloplasmin is the copper-binding protein with a serum level of 200–400mg/litre in adults and children (1–10 years) and 120–300mg/litre in infants and adolescents (10–15 years). Serum copper and caeruloplasmin are reduced in Wilson's disease (hepato-lenticular degeneration), the copper usually being less than 2µmol/litre. Low levels also occur when serum proteins are reduced, as in starvation and nephrosis. Increased levels are caused by pregnancy, the pill, oestrogens, leukaemia and infections. 5ml of clotted blood are required for the estimation of copper and caeruloplasmin.

CORTISOL (Hydrocortisone)

See Plasma 'Cortisol', p. 190, under Blood Tests for Steroids.

C-REACTIVE PROTEIN (CRP)

This is an abnormal protein which appears in the blood during the active phase of many diseases. The results are expressed as 0, 1 +, 2 +, 3 +, 4 + and 5 +. The normal is usually 0 or occasionally 1 +. Raised values occur in bacterial infections, rheumatic fever, myocardial infarction and widespread malignant disease, corresponding roughly to the ESR. It is probably most useful as a guide to rheumatic activity.

CREATINE

Creatine is present in muscles and is necessary for muscle contraction. Normally 175–600µmol/litre (2–7mg/100ml) of creatine is present in blood. Although it is raised in hyperthyroidism and muscular dystrophy blood creatine estimation is now seldom undertaken. For hyperthyroidism see thyroid function tests (pp. 183–7) and for muscular dystrophy see enzymes, especially creatine phosphokinase (p. 92) and creatine in urine (p. 171).

CREATININE

Creatinine is a waste product from creatine. Creatine is necessary for muscle contraction. Normally serum contains 50–100μmol/litre (0.6–1.2mg/100ml) of creatinine in men and 50–80μmol/litre (0.6–0.9mg/100ml) in women. It is excreted through the glomeruli of the kidney and the blood level is a useful index of their function. The blood creatinine rises in kidney diseases when a sufficient number of glomeruli are damaged, and is later to rise than the blood urea. A blood creatinine of over 420μmol/litre (5mg/100ml) in chronic nephritis is of serious significance.

CYCLIC AMP (ADENOSINE MONOPHOSPHATE)

The normal plasma level of cyclic AMP is 12–20nmol/litre. The main clinical value of its estimation is in the diagnosis of hypoparathyroidism. In this condition the plasma level rises to peak values about 20 minutes after injection of parathormone. This does not occur in pseudo-hypoparathyroidism. The laboratory should be contacted for details of the test.

DIGOXIN

Digoxin estimation is performed in cases of suspected digoxin intoxication. 10ml of clotted blood is required, collected at least 6 hours after the last dose. A concentration of up to 2–5nmol/litre is within the accepted therapeutic range. Over 3.8nmol/litre is associated with digoxin toxicity.

DRUGS

The serum level of many drugs can be estimated; this is of particular importance in a suspected overdose. The laboratory should be given detailed information of the drug(s) suspected. The list of drugs which can be assayed is long. It includes anticonvulsants, barbiturates, benzodiazepines, tricyclic antidepressants, cardiac drugs, anti-tubercle drugs and many others. 10ml clotted blood should be sent to the laboratory. The time required varies from 15 minutes to 2 hours, depending on the drug, except for isoniazid which takes 6 hours to assay. In cases of suspected overdose, urine and stomach contents should also be sent where relevant, but should not delay submission of the blood sample (see p. 250).

Electrolytes

Electrolytes are the chemical substances called salts. For example, common salt is sodium chloride. It consists of positively charged sodium ions and negatively charged chloride ions. When it is dissolved in water these ions dissociate and move about almost independently. In blood the two chief electrically positive ions (cations) are sodium and potassium; the two chief electrically negative ions (anions) are chloride and bicarbonate (measured as carbon dioxide or CO_2). These are the substances usually estimated when an electrolyte investigation is requested. They are normally present in the following amounts:

Average Normal Values		*Normal Range*
Sodium	140mmol/litre	133–146mmol/litre
Chloride	100mmol/litre	96–106mmol/litre
Potassium	4mmol/litre	3.5–5.5mmol/litre
Bicarbonate (CO_2)	25mmol/litre (adults)	23–31mmol/litre
	20mmol/litre (children)	18–23mmol/litre

The result is given in millimoles per litre. This is a method of expressing the actual proportions of the different substances present. For the blood electrolytes the figures are numerically the same as those for milli-equivalents per litre, the units recently used.

Electrolyte estimation is of great value in dehydration

from diarrhoea, vomiting, burns or excessive sweating; oedema from kidney failure, heart failure or other causes; diabetic ketosis, Addison's disease and other endocrine disturbances; and also in the control of steroid therapy. Electrolyte estimation is not only a guide as to the treatment to be adopted but later estimations are also a check on the effectiveness of the treatment. It must be emphasised however that mere correction of the electrolyte disturbance in a condition such as intestinal obstruction is of little value unless the obstruction is also relieved by operation. But used in conjunction with treatment of the cause, correction of the electrolyte disturbance can be life-saving.

For electrolyte estimation, 10ml of blood should be placed in a heparin container and sent to the laboratory without delay. A wet syringe or container, or squirting the blood through a fine needle, can haemolyse the blood and make the potassium estimation unreliable. Delay in sending the specimen to the laboratory leads to erroneous results.

WATER AND ELECTROLYTE BALANCE

Water forms 70–90 per cent of our diet, even apparently solid foods consisting largely of water. The normal daily intake for an adult is about 2.5 litres of water, with a minimum total requirement of 1.5 litres. We also eat daily about 5 grams of sodium chloride, of which only half is salt added during cooking and flavouring, and 2–3 grams of potassium, which is found in meat, tea and fruit.

Approximately 70 per cent of the body, by weight, consists of water (75 per cent in children). In a man of 70kg this represents about 50 litres. Water within the cells forms half the body weight (about 35 litres). Water in the plasma is about 3.5 litres and the remainder is in the tissue spaces surrounding the cells. The tissue space fluid and the plasma together are known as extracellular fluid which measures about 15 litres (20 per cent of the body weight). The electrolyte level in the serum or plasma is the same as that in the tissue space fluid.

Dehydration results when 5 per cent of the body weight is lost as water, i.e. about 3 litres for an adult. Twice this loss may be fatal. The fluid loss is mainly from the tissue spaces, with some loss from the plasma which causes haemoconcentration, reflected by raised haemoglobin (p. 45) and haematocrit (p. 47) readings.

When the water content of the body decreases the electrolyte levels tend to rise; when it increases they tend to fall and oedema tends to occur. Often, however, water loss is associated with electrolyte loss. Thus in severe sweating or vomiting there is much loss of chloride. If the fluid lost is replaced by water alone the chloride level in serum and tissue fluid falls. The importance of maintaining the balance between water and electrolytes is thus clear.

In the management of patients with dehydration or oedema, accurate measurement of all fluid intake and output is essential. This is a duty which largely falls to the nurse. It may also be necessary to check salt intake and sometimes output as well. Investigations of value are the plasma or serum osmolality, electrolytes, blood urea, haematocrit and possibly measurement of extracellular fluid volume.

OSMOLALITY (TONICITY)

This is the osmotic pressure produced by all the substances dissolved in the blood. The normal level is 285–295 milliosmol/kg. It is increased in dehydration, e.g. from burns and decreased in water retention, e.g. in pre-eclampsia. By repeating the test after pitressin the distinction between pituitary and renal diabetes insipidus may be made (see also p. 201). Only a small sample of clotted blood or plasma is required. The heparinised blood supplied for electrolytes suffices for osmolality as well.

MEASUREMENT OF FLUID VOLUMES

The volume of the plasma, extracellular water and total body water can be measured by dilution techniques, using suitable chemical or radioactive substances.

A measured dose of the chosen substance is administered, e.g. radioactive bromide by mouth for extracellular fluid volume or Evans blue intravenously for plasma volume. After sufficient time for complete distribution, a blood sample is collected. The amount of substance present is estimated. From the degree of dilution, the extracellular fluid volume or the plasma volume can be calculated. These methods are used in certain centres for investigating dehydration, oedema, malnutrition and obesity.

Enzymes

Enzymes are substances which promote chemical reactions in the body. When cells are damaged, their enzymes escape into the body fluids and tend to raise the blood level above normal values. It should be noted that the normal values tend to vary from one laboratory to another, depending on the reagents and temperatures used. It is therefore recommended that the values quoted are checked against the local normal values. For each test about 5ml of clotted blood is required.

ALDOLASE

Normal range is 0–6iu/litre. Raised values occur in all types of tissue damage, e.g. muscle, heart and liver. It is non-specific and now little used. Haemolysis invalidates the result.

AMINOTRANSFERASES (TRANSAMINASES)

Two types of aminotransferase are usually estimated. One is Aspartate Transferase (AST) (Serum Glutamic

Oxalacetic Transaminase, SGOT) with a normal level of 5–35iu/litre in adults and up to 100iu/litre in children. The other is Alanine Aminotransferase (ALT) (Serum Glutamic Pyruvic Transaminase, SGPT) with a normal level of 5–28iu/litre in adults and up to 75iu/litre in children. Increase occurs in acute liver damage, in heart muscle damage due to coronary artery disease and in skeletal muscle damage from injury or disease. In acute liver disease both types are increased, up to 1 000iu/litre or more (see pp. 21–2). In heart muscle damage the increase mainly affects Aspartate Transferase (AST), up to 100–200iu/litre or more, but only lasting a few days. This is very helpful when the clinical and ECG changes are doubtful, when samples should be collected on three successive days.

AMYLASE (see p. 25)

CHOLINESTERASE (PSEUDOCHOLINESTERASE)

This enzyme is necessary for nervous tissue to return to normal after it has been stimulated. The normal level is 2.6–5.3iu/litre in males and 1.9–4.6iu/litre in females. In some families this enzyme is present in smaller amounts and in an unusual form. This results in delayed recovery of normal respiration after anaesthesia in which a muscle relaxant (suxamethonium) has been used. Such delayed postoperative recovery is an indication for cholinesterase estimation in the patient and blood relatives.

An acquired form of cholinesterase deficiency can occur after exposure to certain pesticides and phosphate-rich fertilisers, leading to general lethargy.

CREATINE PHOSPHOKINASE (CPK)

Normal range is 0–85iu/litre in males and 0–60iu/litre in females, with higher values in children. Exercise increases the values, so the patient must be at rest for 2 hours before collection. After 6–36 hours abnormal increase occurs in muscle damage, degeneration and dystrophy.

GAMMA GLUTAMYL TRANSFERASE (TRANSPEPTIDASE), γ GT

This enzyme provides a very sensitive indicator of all types of liver disease, the serum level being raised when there is damage to liver cells. The normal range is 10–45iu/litre in men and 10–35iu/litre in women. It is always raised in alcoholics, even when there is no other evidence of liver damage. It is also raised in pancreatic disease and in 50 per cent of patients with cardiac infarction. It is not raised in bone disease and so can assist in determining the cause for a raised serum alkaline phosphatase.

ISOCITRIC DEHYDROGENASE (ICDH)

The normal level is up to 7iu/litre. It is most useful in the differential diagnosis of liver disease. In acute viral hepatitis the values are 10–20 times normal. In obstructive jaundice or cholestatic hepatosis the levels are only slightly increased. Intermediate values are seen in cirrhosis of the liver and tumour deposits, also with placental degeneration in pre-eclamptic toxaemia. Any haemolysis of the specimen invalidates the result. The enzyme may also be estimated on CSF (see p. 130).

LACTIC DEHYDROGENASE (LDH)

Lactic dehydrogenase levels provide a measure of the extent of tissue damage. The normal level is 70 to 240iu/litre. It is increased in myocardial infarction 36 hours to 6 days after the onset of pain. The increase is proportional to the extent of the infarction. With values of over 1 000iu/litre the outcome is often fatal. Raised levels also occur in carcinoma with secondary deposits, especially in the liver, in leukaemia, haemolytic anaemia (including sickle cell), pernicious anaemia, muscular dystrophy and in some chronic renal diseases. Haemolysis of the specimen invalidates the result.

α-HYDROXYBUTYRATE DEHYDROGENASE (HBD)

The normal level is 0–140iu/litre. This enzyme forms part of the LDH complex and is LDH-1-isoenzyme. It occurs chiefly in the heart, kidneys and red cells, so it is a more specific test for myocardial infarction than total LDH. Like LDH, haemolysis of the sample must be avoided.

5-NUCLEOTIDASE

Estimation of this enzyme is of value when there is a raised serum alkaline phosphatase (p. 83) for which the cause is uncertain. 5-Nucleotidase serum level is raised in liver disease, but not in bone disease, the normal level being 2–15iu/litre.

PHOSPHATASES (see p. 83)

FERRITIN

Ferritin is a protein containing iron. The normal serum level is 10–250μg/litre. It is reduced in iron deficiency and increased when there is iron overload, as in haemochromatosis or in patients who have had multiple transfusions, e.g. for Mediterranean anaemia. For its estimation 10ml of clotted blood is required. It provides a means of assessing the total iron storage in the body, 1μg/litre of serum ferritin being approximately equivalent to 8mg of storage iron in the body. False high values can occur in liver diseases. This investigation is not yet available in all hospital laboratories.

α-FETOPROTEIN (AFP, see p. 81)

Normal adult serum contains virtually no α-fetoprotein. It is present in about half the cases of liver carcinoma (hepatoma). It is also present in some cases of gastro-intestinal cancer and occasionally in lung cancer.

FIBRINOGEN (see p. 55)

GASTRIN (see p. 18)

GLUCOSE (see sugar, p. 102)

GLUCOSE TOLERANCE TEST (see p. 29)

INSULIN (see serum insulin, p. 31)

IRON

For the following tests 10–20ml of clotted blood are required. It must be collected with an iron-free syringe (a plastic disposable syringe appears satisfactory) into a specially prepared iron-free container.

Serum Iron
The normal value is 1–3mmol/litre (60–180μg/ml). Low figures are found in the iron deficiency anaemias, scurvy and polycythaemia. Raised levels occur in infective hepatitis (see p. 23) and in haemochromatosis.

Iron-binding Capacity
The iron in serum is bound to a protein. This measures the maximum amount of iron with which the protein can combine. Normally it is 4.5–8mmol/litre (250–450μg/ml). It is increased in iron deficiency.

Iron Saturation
This is calculated from the above results. It is the proportion of iron actually present compared to the total iron-binding capacity, expressed as a percentage. Normally it is 15–50 per cent. In iron deficiency it is usually less than 10 per cent. In pernicious anaemia and haemochromatosis it is usually nearly 100 per cent.

LITHIUM

The use of lithium carbonate in the treatment of depression is controlled by the estimation of serum lithium, the accepted therapeutic range being 0.6–1.2mmol/litre. 10ml of clotted blood is required, collected at least 3 hours after the last dose.

LIVER FUNCTION TESTS (see pp. 19–24)

PARACETAMOL

In cases of paracetamol overdose the blood level of the drug determines whether treatment with an antidote is necessary. Four hours after the overdose or as soon as possible thereafter, 10ml of blood is taken into a heparin container and sent to the Chemical Pathology (Clinical Biochemistry) department for urgent estimation of the blood paracetamol level. The result is plotted on a graph (Fig. 2/1), and the area in which it falls determines the treatment.

NB The graph outlines the procedure currently followed in Bristol and Cardiff but there are regional variations.

PARATHORMONE

Parathormone is the hormone secreted by the parathyroid glands. Its action is to raise the serum calcium. Serum parathormone is increased in tumours of the parathyroid gland and renal osteodystrophy. It may be reduced as a result of accidental surgical removal of the parathyroid glands during thyroidectomy. In some centres the serum parathormone level can now be measured.

PHENYLALANINE

By estimating the blood level of phenylalanine on all babies at the age of one week it is possible to detect phenyl-

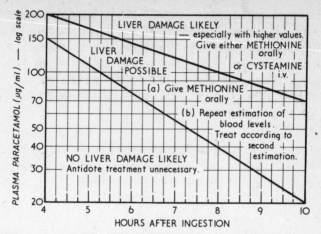

Fig. 2/1   Management of paracetamol overdose. Liver damage related to paracetamol and number of hours

ketonuria (PKU) before the brain is damaged. Using Guthrie's test, a few drops of blood are collected on to thick filter paper from a heel-prick, the collection usually being done by the district nurse. The amount of phenylalanine is measured by the amount of bacterial growth (B. subtilis) that it promotes. (In some laboratories this test is now being replaced by a chemical method.) Normal blood contains less than 0.25mmol/litre (4mg/100ml). A level greater than this requires further investigation.

Phenylalanine is present in all food protein. In phenyl-ketonuria the liver lacks an enzyme needed to control the blood level of phenylalanine and it rises, e.g. to 1mmol/litre (16mg/100ml) and above. This leads to mental deficiency unless treatment is started very early in life.

PHOSPHORUS AND PHOSPHATASES (see p. 83)

PROGESTERONE

Blood progesterone may be estimated in the investigation of female infertility. Normally the blood level rises during the latter half of the menstrual cycle. If infertility is due to failure of ovulation the normal rise does not occur. One sample is taken on the 8–10th day and a second sample on the 20–23rd day of the menstrual cycle: 5ml blood is collected into a lithium heparin tube and placed in the refrigerator until it can be taken to the laboratory.

PROTEINS

About 5ml of blood are sent to the laboratory in a dry tube, for the estimation of serum proteins. The total proteins are 60–80g/litre (6–8g/100ml) of which 33–55g/litre (3.5–5.5g/100ml) is albumin and 15–33g/litre (1.5–3.3g/100ml) is globulin.

Where the plasma proteins are requested the blood must be sent in a Sequestrene or heparin container. The only difference from the serum proteins is the addition of fibrinogen, this being normally 2–4g/litre (0.2–0.4g/100ml). Fibrinogen is usually estimated on its own. (See p. 55.)

The albumin is diminished in liver and kidney diseases; the globulin is increased in liver diseases and to a much greater extent in multiple myeloma and kala-azar. In starvation both albumin and globulin are diminished.

PROTEIN ELECTROPHORESIS

Separation of the serum protein into its various components may be carried out by electrophoresis. The passage of an electric current causes the different protein components to move at different speeds along a cellulose acetate strip, causing them to separate from each other. The globulin is separated into four parts called α_1, α_2, β and γ-globulin. The abnormal γ-globulin in multiple myeloma may be shown by this method, also the deficiency of γ-globulin in agammaglobulinaemia. Electrophoresis may also be performed using filter paper, starch gel or a starch block instead of cellulose acetate.

IMMUNOGLOBULINS

These are globulins concerned with immunity, i.e. anti-bodies. Their estimation involves the use of a specific anti-body against each immunoglobulin. That with the largest molecules is called macroglobulin or IgM (Immuno-globulin M); the normal serum level is 0.5–2.0g/litre (50–200mg/100ml). Gamma(γ) globulin is IgG (Immunoglobulin G); its normal serum level is 6–16g/litre (0.6–1.6g/100ml). Other immunoglobulins are IgA, IgD and IgE. Excessive and abnormal (monoclonal) IgG is produced in myelomatosis and excessive IgM in macro-globulinaemia.

IgE can now be estimated by the SAS. The adult serum level is 0–840 (mean 95) U/ml with lower levels in children. It is raised in many allergic conditions, particularly those with an immediate hypersensitivity reaction, e.g. asthma. The expensive RAST (Radio-Allergo-Sorbent Test) is rarely positive if serum IgE is less than 300U/ml.

Immune Paresis Studies are undertaken by the SAS when immune response is impaired, either as a congenital defect or secondary, e.g. to lymphoma or nephrosis. About 10ml clotted blood and a 24-hour urine are required. Clinical history and details of vaccination by, e.g. tetanus toxoid, polio vaccine, BCG and Mantoux response must be given.

PYRUVIC ACID

Normally the blood pyruvic acid is 0.045–0.110mmol/litre (0.4–1.0mg/100ml). In vitamin B_1 deficiency it may be increased up to 0.22–0.33mmol/litre (2–3mg/100ml) and is used as a test for this condition. Some increase also occurs in diabetes mellitus, congestive heart failure and other conditions. The blood is usually collected by one of the laboratory staff.

PYRUVIC TOLERANCE TEST

This is a more sensitive test for vitamin B_1 deficiency than simple blood pyruvic acid level determination. The laboratory staff must be notified and may undertake the blood collection. The test is performed in the morning, the patient having fasted since 22.00h the previous evening (water may be drunk). A 2ml fasting blood sample is collected. Then 50g of glucose is given orally in about 300ml of water flavoured with diabetic squash. Further 2ml blood samples are collected at $\frac{1}{2}$, 1 and 2 hours after the glucose. Special care is required for blood collection. The syringe must not be warm. Either a 2ml or 5ml syringe is used with a 21-gauge needle. The patient must not clench and unclench the hand. The tourniquet is kept on for the minimum of time, being removed immediately after the needle enters the vein. The 2ml of blood is ejected into 8ml of cold trichloracetic acid in a stoppered centrifuge tube. The blood pyruvic acid level should not exceed 0.132mmol/litre (1.2mg/100ml) for any specimen. In vitamin B_1 deficiency this level is exceeded.

REACTION (pH) AND BLOOD GASES

The pH of the blood is the degree of acidity or alkalinity. This can be measured by means of an instrument called a pH meter. A pH of 7 is neutral. Increase in the pH above 7 corresponds to an increase in alkalinity. Decrease below 7 corresponds to an increase in acidity.

For this test 2–5ml of very fresh heparinised blood are usually needed, collected with a heparinised syringe. With the newer pH meters a finger-prick sample will suffice. Normal blood is slightly alkaline, having a pH of 7.35 to 7.42. The body maintains this pH at the stable level necessary for life by means of buffer systems; one of the most important is the bicarbonate/CO_2 system. Bicarbonate is controlled by the kidneys (metabolic) and CO_2 by the lungs (respiratory). Only when the buffer systems break down does the pH fall outside the normal range. In acidosis, e.g. diabetic coma or respiratory distress, the pH may fall below 7.35. In alkalosis, e.g. from severe vomiting or excessive alkali therapy, the pH may be increased above 7.42.

The pH meter may also be used to measure the carbon dioxide pressure (pCO_2) and oxygen pressure (pO_2) in blood, also the standard bicarbonate and base excess. The normal values are as follows:

Carbon dioxide pressure (pCO_2)	34–45mmHg
Oxygen pressure (pO_2)	80–110mmHg
Standard bicarbonate	21.3–24.8mmol/litre
Base excess	−2.3 to +2.3mmol/litre

In respiratory distress the pCO_2 is increased and the pO_2 reduced; the standard bicarbonate, the base excess and the pH are also all reduced. Other combinations of these findings give a measure of the severity of respiratory or metabolic acidosis or alkalosis.

For these estimations anaerobically collected fresh heparinised arterial blood is required, normally collected by the medical officer using a heparinised syringe. The laboratory will collect arterialised capillary blood in non-cyanotic cases. In adults the hand is placed in water at 45°C (just above body temperature) for about 5 minutes immediately before the blood is collected. The sample must be analysed within half an hour of collection.

RENIN-ANGIOTENSIN SYSTEM

In cases of hypertension where there is evidence of possible unilateral kidney disease, revealed for example by IVP (p. 219), it is feasible to collect blood for renin-angiotensin estimation from each renal vein to see whether excess is being produced by one kidney compared to the other. This assists in deciding whether surgical removal of a damaged kidney may relieve hypertension. For this test 5–20ml of blood are collected into a universal container to which a special enzyme inhibitor has been added. The collection is usually carried out by a radiologist after he has introduced a catheter from the femoral vein into the inferior vena cava. Prior to the test all drugs are stopped, particularly hypotensive drugs. Sometimes a diuretic is given on the morning of the test to exaggerate any renin-angiotensin difference between the two kidneys.

SUGAR (Glucose)

The normal fasting glucose for whole blood is 3.6–5.6mmol/litre (65–100mg/100ml) for adults and 2.2–5.6mmol/litre (40–100mg/100ml) for children. For this estimation 2ml of blood is taken into a fluoride bottle. The fasting glucose for plasma is slightly higher, being 4.2–6.0mmol/litre (75–107mg/100ml). For this estimation 5ml of blood is taken into a heparin tube. In diabetes mellitus the blood sugar as a whole is higher than normal and may rise to over 28mmol/litre (500mg/100ml). Estimation of the blood sugar is of the greatest importance in diabetes, and is a guide to the diet to be given and the amount of insulin required. It is an essential part of the satisfactory treatment of diabetic coma.

It is important to know how long has elapsed since a meal. A 'fasting' blood sugar is frequently taken.

The blood sugar is also of considerable importance in the diagnosis of 'spontaneous hypoglycaemia' when the blood sugar falls below normal limits due to the action of insulin. The estimation also enables other conditions (renal glycosuria, absorption of breast milk, etc.) which give rise to reducing substances in the urine to be distinguished from diabetes.

A further modification of blood sugar estimation—the glucose tolerance test—is described elsewhere (p. 29).

Approximate Blood Sugar Estimation may be obtained in the ward or casualty department by means of Dextrostix. A large drop of blood is spread on the printed side of the test strip. After exactly 1 minute it is washed off with a jet of cold water and the colour compared with the chart provided. A more accurate estimation is obtained by measuring the colour with a reflectance meter.

TRANSAMINASES (AMINOTRANSFERASES) (see p. 91)

TRIGLYCERIDES

Triglycerides are the neutral fats, carried by the blood in the form of chylomicrons (microscopic fatty droplets), and lipoproteins. The normal range is up to 2.1mmol/litre in men and up to 1.6mmol/litre in women. Raised values are found in most cases of hyperlipoproteinaemia which may be familiar or due to a metabolic disorder, e.g. diabetes mellitus. People with raised serum triglycerides are likely to develop atherosclerosis and ischaemic heart disease. Five basic types of hyperlipoproteinaemia have been distinguished by electrophoresis.

UREA

Urea is the main end product of protein breakdown. The normal figure for blood urea is 2.5–7.5mmol/litre (15–45mg/100ml) with higher values in old people.

2ml of clotted blood or a finger-prick specimen is sufficient. A quick ward test (Azostix) is described on p. 156. When kidney function is sufficiently impaired the blood urea rises, the condition being called uraemia.

In uraemia the figure may be raised considerably to 33mmol/litre (200mg/100ml), 50mmol/litre (300mg/100ml) or even 100mmol/litre (600mg/100ml). If over 50mmol/litre the case is often fatal, though not necessarily so.

In surgical cases the estimation is of value in considering the question of operation on the genito-urinary system, e.g. prostate cases and renal cases. About 8mmol/litre

(48mg/100ml) or more in a patient with hypertrophy of the prostate may indicate the advisability of the operation being done in two stages. The blood urea also rises considerably in cases of:

1. Gastro-intestinal lesions with obstruction or haemorrhage.

2. Severe shock, especially following crushing injuries, burns and obstetrical conditions, e.g. eclampsia.

URIC ACID

The normal figure is 0.15–0.4mmol/litre (2.5–7mg/100ml) for men and 0.1–0.35mmol/litre (1.5–6mg/100ml) for women. About 5ml of blood are sent to the laboratory in either a dry or a sequestrenated tube.

In eclampsia the figure may be 0.3mmol/litre (5mg/100ml) to 0.36mmol/litre (6mg/100ml). In gout it may rise as high as 0.6mmol/litre (10mg/100ml).

SECTION THREE
The Cardiovascular System

The Cardiovascular System

The blood pressure is the pressure the blood exerts on the wall of the blood vessel. The arterial blood pressure is the one commonly recorded. It is expressed as a figure which indicates the height in millimetres of a column of mercury (mmHg) that would be supported by the pressure in question. It is estimated by means of a sphygmomanometer containing a column of mercury to which is attached a millimetre scale. A cuff is placed around the upper arm which can be inflated by means of a rubber bulb, and it is attached to the manometer by a length of rubber tubing. Other types of sphygmomanometer are available which record on a spring principle, with a gauge like a watch. These types are not so accurate or reliable as the mercurial column.

There are two readings to be taken in measuring the blood pressure:

Systolic. The pressure corresponding to systole, or contraction of the ventricle of the heart.
Diastolic. The pressure corresponding to diastole, or relaxation of the ventricle.

The simplest way to take the blood pressure is to feel the pulse at the wrist, inflate the armband, and note the figure reading of the mercury at which the pulse disappears.

It is, however, desirable to record both systolic and diastolic pressures, and for this purpose a stethoscope is placed over the brachial artery in the region of the elbow. Air is pumped into the armlet till no sounds are audible. The pressure is then allowed to fall slowly by opening the valve. At the point when regular sounds become audible, a reading is taken—this is the systolic pressure. The pressure is still allowed to fall, and the sounds change in character, ultimately becoming practically inaudible, when another reading is taken—this is the diastolic pressure.

The difference between the two readings is termed the pulse pressure. Normal systolic blood pressure may vary from 100 to 140mmHg. It tends to increase with age. Normal diastolic pressure varies from 60 to 90mmHg. A blood pressure reading is usually expressed thus: 120/90, 210/140, etc. This indicates that the systolic pressure is 120 and the diastolic 90, and so on.

A high blood pressure is found in cases of essential hypertension, chronic renal disease, cerebral compression, toxaemias of pregnancy, etc. A low blood pressure (hypotension) is found in cases of haemorrhage, shock, severe acute infections, Addison's disease, etc, when the systolic blood pressure may fall below 90mmHg.

Estimation of the blood pressure is one of the commonest of all tests, and is carried out on the majority of patients.

CENTRAL VENOUS PRESSURE (CVP)

This is the pressure in the large veins returning blood to the heart. It is normally between −20mm (−2cm) and +80mm (+8cm) of water. It is raised in heart failure or following excessive intravenous infusion. It is low in dehydration and following haemorrhage. There are also fluctuations with respiration and pulsations with the heart beat.

The pressure is measured by a CVP line. This is a fine plastic catheter inserted aseptically, usually via the arm, and long enough to place the tip in the superior vena cava close to the heart. The other end is connected via a three-way tap to a sterile manometer set and a standard 'drip' set with a suitable infusion fluid. When taking a measurement, a spirit level is used to align the sternal notch of the patient with the zero point on the manometer. The CVP line is of particular value when the intravenous fluid requirements are uncertain.

APICAL HEART RATE

With a stethoscope over the apex of the heart two heart sounds—'lub-dup'—are normally heard for each heart beat. It is advisable to count the heart rate in this way in heart conditions such as atrial fibrillation where some heart impulses fail to reach the radial pulse.

ARRHYTHMIA MONITORING

Many units for the intensive care of cardiac patients now have an arrhythmia monitor. This is an electronic apparatus with electrodes which are attached to the patient. The instrument can then monitor the heart rate and ECG. It detects any change in the heart rhythm, recording it automatically and warning the staff so that appropriate treatment can be given at an early stage, e.g. by a defibrillator.

CARDIAC CATHETERISATION (including angiocardiography)

For this test full aseptic precautions are essential.

A cardiac catheter, usually made of polythene tubing, is introduced into a vein, generally in the left cubital fossa. Its progress is watched under x-rays until it is seen to enter the heart. Blood is then withdrawn from the pulmonary artery, right ventricle, right atrium and superior vena cava. Blood pressures may also be measured at these sites. The samples of blood removed are examined for their oxygen and carbon dioxide content. Normally these remain practically the same in all the samples. Where there is a short circuit between the left and right sides of the heart, a marked rise in the oxygen content will be found to occur when the catheter has reached the site of the defect, e.g. right atrium in atrial septal defect.

Angiocardiography. This is the injection of radio-opaque dye through the catheter, so that by means of x-rays many abnormalities of the heart structure can be demonstrated. A cine-film is often taken (cine-radiography).

Coronary Angiography is a similar technique for outlining the coronary arteries. It is used in conjunction with the exercise tolerance test (p. 112) to assess coronary artery sufficiency before undertaking a cardiac bypass.

Cardiac catheterisation is chiefly of value in the investigation of any heart disease where surgery is contemplated, including congenital heart disease. The preparation of the patient prior to this investigation is important. Penicillin therapy is started on the day of operation. A suitable sedative is given 1 hour before. The penicillin is continued for 2 days following the operation.

ECHOCARDIOGRAPHY

An ultrasound beam is directed at the heart. Movement of the heart walls and of individual valves is detected by the Doppler principle. The record may be displayed on a screen or on paper. It is used in the diagnosis of valve disease and pericardial effusion.

ELECTROCARDIOGRAM (ECG)

Electrical disturbances are set up by cardiac contractions, and these may be recorded in the form of a graphic chart, an electrocardiogram, or displayed on an ECG monitor. Wires from the ECG machine are attached to the patient's limbs and chest, and transmit electrical impulses from the patient's heart to the machine.

The ECG records the electrical changes associated with atrial contraction (P wave), passage of the impulse from atria to ventricles (PR interval), ventricular contraction (QRS complex) and ventricular repolarisation (T wave) (Fig. 3/1). If there is atrial fibrillation the P wave is no

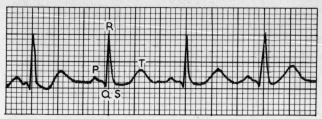

Fig. 3/1   Normal ECG

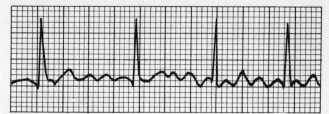

Fig. 3/2   Atrial fibrillation

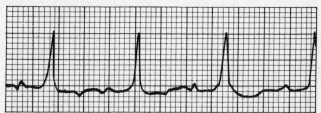

Fig. 3/3   Partial heart block

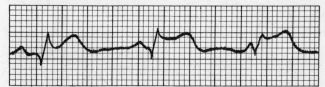

Fig. 3/4   Myocardial infarction

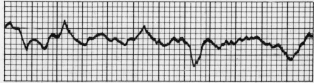

Fig. 3/5   Ventricular fibrillation

longer produced (Fig. 3/2). If conduction from atria to ventricles is slowed by partial heart block, the length of the PR interval is prolonged (Fig. 3/3). If the ventricular muscle is damaged, as in myocardial infarction due to coronary thrombosis, the pattern of the ST segment and/or T wave is altered (Fig. 3/4).

Now that cardiac monitoring is a routine on intensive care wards, it is necessary to become familiar with the normal ECG and to distinguish between a trivial abnormality such as an atrial ectopic beat and a major disaster such as ventricular fibrillation (Fig. 3/5).

EXERCISE TOLERANCE TEST

This is a method of estimating the reserve power of the heart in cases of cardiac disease.

The patient is given some definite amount of physical effort to carry out, e.g. walking a certain distance, climbing a certain number of steps, stepping on and off a stool several times, etc, and the effect on the heart is noted. The pulse rate is taken before the test, immediately following exercise and again after a rest of 2 minutes. If the reserve power of the heart is sufficient for the task in question, the pulse rate should not be unduly increased by the exercise, and should have returned to its original rate after the 2 minutes' rest.

Another method of estimating the reserve power of the heart is to see how much physical effort the patient can carry out without developing any signs of cardiac distress, e.g. severe palpitation, shortness of breath, faintness or pain.

PHONOCARDIOGRAM

The heart sounds may be recorded graphically. This is carried out by means of a special instrument called a phonocardiograph. By this means it is possible to detect and record heart sounds which are inaudible or difficult to distinguish by the ear. By means of an electrocardiogram recorded simultaneously it is possible to correlate the heart sounds with the heart action. It is of value in the interpretation of heart murmurs.

SECTION FOUR
The Respiratory System

The Respiratory System

RHINOSCOPY

This is the examination of the interior of the nose.

Anterior rhinoscopy is carried out through the nostrils with the aid of a nasal speculum and good illumination.

Posterior rhinoscopy is the examination of the naso-pharnyx which is carried out through the mouth with the aid of a reflecting mirror (warmed, e.g. with a spirit lamp) or else with a pharyngoscope. The patient's pharynx is sprayed with local anaesthetic to permit vision behind the soft palate. No food is permitted until recovery from the anaesthesia. Swabs may be taken for bacteriology or tissue for histology (taken into fixative, e.g. formalin).

NASAL SWAB

One of the following techniques is normally used:

1. Swab from anterior nares (nostrils). Using a sterile bacterial swab, material is collected from just within the anterior nares. This is the method of choice in the detection of staphylococcus carriers, where swabs should also be taken from wrists, perineum and groin.
2. Per-nasal swab. See below.

PER-NASAL SWAB

This swab is supplied by the laboratory. It is supported on a thin flexible metal wire. It is introduced through the anterior nares and passed directly posteriorly along the floor of the nose, until the posterior nasopharynx is reached. Care must be taken to choose the side of the nose which is free from any obstruction, e.g. by septal deflection. This method is used in suspected infections by meningococcus, bordetella pertussis (whooping cough) and nasal diphtheria. The swab should be sent to the laboratory in a transport medium (see p. 230).

THROAT SWABS

Sterile swabs are supplied by the laboratory. The patient is placed so that the pharynx is well illuminated. If necessary the tongue may be depressed by a spatula. The specimen should be collected by rubbing the swab firmly over the tonsillar area. If a membrane is present, this should be lifted gently, and the swab taken from the deeper layers. Gargling with antiseptics, or drinking hot fluids, should be avoided for an hour or so prior to taking the swab.

Diphtheria Bacilli
In all cases of throat infection a swab should be sent to the laboratory. If the case is diphtheria the result will be 'Diphtheria bacilli present' or '+ve for KLB' (KLB=Klebs Löffler bacillus—the cause of diphtheria). A repeated negative result usually means the case is not one of diphtheria.

Swab results are also useful in assessing when a convalescent case of diphtheria is clear of infection.

'Carriers'
Some persons, whether convalescent from diphtheria or not, carry diphtheria bacilli in their throats when perfectly well, and they may be a source of infection to others. In such cases a 'virulence' test is done to decide whether the bacteria present are capable of causing diphtheria or not. If 'virulent' the patient must be isolated until clear of infection. If 'non-virulent' they may be disregarded.

Nasal swabs and aural swabs may also be taken from patients who have a chronic discharge, and who may be potential carriers of diphtheria.

Streptococci
Many persons harbour streptococci in the throat which may

or may not be harmful to others. The ones most liable to cause trouble are 'haemolytic streptococci', i.e. those capable of haemolysing blood. These are especially dangerous to maternity cases, and may cause puerperal sepsis.

Anyone working in a maternity ward who has a sore throat·should have a throat swab and nasal swab taken. Clinical staff with a throat swab 'positive for haemolytic streptococci' must be excluded until three negative results have been obtained. It may be necessary for carriers of streptococci to have the tonsils removed.

Vincent's Angina
In cases of this disease a throat or gum swab will reveal the presence of the causal organisms, spirochaetes and fusiform bacilli.

LARYNGOSCOPY

This investigation may be carried out in two ways.

1. Indirect vision

The patient is seated on a chair in a darkened room. A beam of light is directed from a reflecting mirror on the operator's forehead into the patient's mouth. The laryngeal mirror is warmed to prevent condensation, care being taken that it does not burn the patient. This is introduced into the mouth just beneath the uvula and adjusted so that the epiglottis and larynx can be viewed. It is chiefly of value for examining the vocal cords for paralysis, infections and growths.

2. Direct vision
A laryngoscope fitted with light is introduced over the back of the tongue, with the patient's neck extended over a pillow. A direct view of the larynx can be obtained in this way. This method is most commonly used by anaesthetists introducing laryngeal tubes during anaesthesia.

BRONCHOSCOPY

By means of a bronchoscope the main bronchi and their branches can be inspected. In addition to the rigid broncho-scope, a flexible fibre-optic instrument is now available. No food is taken for several hours before this procedure is carried out. A sedative is given, and the patient prepared for the theatre. Its chief value is in the diagnosis of growths, and small portions of tissue can be removed for histological examination. It is also used for removing foreign bodies from the air passages.

THORACOSCOPY

After artificial pneumothorax has been induced, the pleura may be inspected with the aid of a thoracoscope. In addition to the diagnosis of disease involving the pleura, it is of value in cutting adhesions which prevent full collapse of the lung.

Laboratory Examination of Sputum

The specimen sent to the laboratory should be freshly expectorated sputum, not saliva or food debris. For suspected malignant cells see Cytology, p. 245.

The following may be found:

Blood is present in any of the conditions giving rise to haemoptysis, e.g. tuberculosis, mitral stenosis, bronchiectasis and growths.
Elastic fibres in cases of lung destruction, e.g. tuberculosis, abscess of lung.
Parasites, e.g. hooklets in hydatid disease.
Pus in acute and chronic inflammation, e.g. pneumonia, bronchiectasis, abscess of lung, etc.
Eosinophils and characteristic mucous plugs in asthma.

BACTERIA

In pneumonia—pneumococci, streptococci, etc. In legionnaire's disease, L. pneumophila can be isolated but requires culture facilities which are only available in certain laboratories.

In bronchitis, asthma, bronchiectasis, abscess of the lung, gangrene of the lung, many different types of bacteria, including anaerobic organisms and fungi may be found.

TUBERCLE BACILLI

In pulmonary tuberculosis, the number of tubercle bacilli in the sputum may be reported as 'few', 'moderate numbers' or 'many'.

If tubercle bacilli are not found on a routine test, they may be demonstrable by a concentration test in which the sputum is centrifuged after digestion with antiformin, the deposit examined microscopically and also inoculated on to culture media. It may also be tested by guinea-pig inoculation. If tubercle bacilli are isolated they are then tested for sensitivity to the appropriate antibiotics.

Gastric Washings

If the sputum is negative on ordinary examination, tubercle bacilli may be found by examination of the gastric juice owing to swallowed sputum, particularly in children. An early morning specimen before breakfast is taken.

A sterile gastric tube is passed and about 100ml of sterile water injected into the stomach. Some 10–15 minutes later this fluid is aspirated, put into a sterile bottle and sent to the laboratory.

Laryngeal Swab

This is a valuable alternative to sputum in adults who are unable to produce sputum. A special swab shaped like a hockey stick is provided by the laboratory. The patient's tongue is held forward with gauze and the swab introduced round the back of the tongue into the larynx. The operator must wear a face mask and gown, and avoid the expiratory gust of the patient's cough.

Pleural Fluid

The fluid is drawn off through an aspirating needle, and sent to the laboratory in a sterile container, preferably with a few drops of sterile 20% sodium citrate as an anti-coagulant (prepared container available from laboratory). Normally no detectable fluid is present in the pleural cavity.

Blood-stained fluid occurs in cases of growths of the lungs, in some injuries of the chest, and occasionally in tuberculosis.

CLEAR FLUID

Containing polymorphs
This is usually the precursor of an empyema.

Containing lymphocytes
This may be tuberculous. (See guinea-pig test p. 123.)

Containing endothelial cells
This is usually an effusion arising from a failing heart.

Malignant cells
Malignant cells may be seen in effusions accompanying growths of the lung.

PURULENT FLUID

In pneumococcal empyema the pus is thick, creamy yellow, and contains numerous pneumococci. In streptococcal empyema, the pus is thinner and contains streptococci. In tuberculous cases the pus is greenish yellow in colour, and tubercle bacilli may be demonstrable. See also Infected Fluids, p. 229.

GUINEA-PIG TEST

In a doubtful case of tuberculosis with a clear effusion where culture for tubercle is negative, some of the fluid can be sent for injection into a guinea-pig.

Lung Function Tests

VITAL CAPACITY OF LUNGS

This is the maximum amount of air which can be expired following a full inspiration. The patient blows through a tube into an inverted jar filled with water. The average is 3 000 to 6 000ml. It varies considerably according to sex, height and general physique. In diseases of the lungs the vital capacity is diminished, sometimes to as little as 500ml.

FORCED EXPIRATORY VOLUME (FEV_1 or Timed Vital Capacity)

This is the maximum volume of air that can be forcibly expired in one second, after full inspiration. It is measured with a special spirometer. Normally it is 3 000–5 000ml in 1 second. It can be greatly reduced by disease even though the vital capacity is normal and depends on the following factors:

1. The freedom of the air passages from obstruction.
2. The elasticity of the lungs.
3. The state of the chest wall, muscles, diaphragm and pleura.

It is reduced in emphysema and in any other disease affecting the above factors. It is the best general test of lung function. (A Vitalograph may be used for VC and FEV_1.)

WRIGHT'S PEAK FLOW METER

This is a machine for measuring the maximum speed of expiration. Normally it is 300–700litres/minute. This figure is reduced if there is airways obstruction from any cause, e.g. chronic bronchitis or asthma.

SECTION FIVE
The Nervous System

X-ray Examinations of Central Nervous System, see p. 222

The Nervous System

Cerebrospinal Fluid

The examination of cerebrospinal fluid is an essential part of the investigation of certain diseases of the nervous system. About 5ml are required for a complete examination, 1ml being placed in a fluoride tube for glucose estimation. The fluid is obtained by lumbar puncture.

LUMBAR PUNCTURE

For this procedure the nurse prepares a sterile trolley containing towels, swabs, spirit, iodine, local anaesthetic with syringe and needles, the special lumbar puncture needles with stilettes, and the manometer with tubing attached. Underneath the trolley there should be two or three sterile universal containers. The patient should be lying on his side with the knees and chin closely approximated. Both the head and buttocks should be at the same level. The puncture is usually made between the spines of the 2nd and 3rd lumbar vertebrae after cleaning and anaesthetising the skin.

PRESSURE OF CEREBROSPINAL FLUID

This is estimated by a manometer which is a calibrated glass tube, attached to the lumbar puncture needle by means of a rubber tube. The height of the fluid in the tube above the level of the needle gives the pressure of the cerebrospinal fluid in millimetres of cerebrospinal fluid. Normally this pressure is 75–150mm of cerebrospinal fluid and is affected by pulse and respiration. Pressure significantly above 150mm indicates an increased intracranial pressure, often due to cerebral tumour or infection.

The estimation of the pressure by observing the rate of flow through the lumbar puncture needle is not reliable.

QUECKENSTEDT'S TEST

Compression of both jugular veins with the manometer in position causes a sharp rise in the cerebrospinal fluid pressure, followed by a sharp fall when the pressure is released. Coughing produces a similar rise and fall. When the flow of the cerebrospinal fluid is obstructed, for instance by a spinal tumour, this rise and fall is diminished in amount and rate. Where the obstruction is complete no rise occurs.

CISTERNAL PUNCTURE

In cases where lumbar puncture is not practicable, cerebrospinal fluid can be obtained by cisternal puncture.

The back of the patient's neck should be shaved and full aseptic precautions are necessary as for lumbar puncture. The patient is seated with the head well flexed and held by an assistant. The skin is anaesthetised and a lumbar puncture needle is introduced through the foramen magnum into the cisterna magna. This method is used in cases of complete spinal block.

Examination of the Cerebrospinal Fluid

ROUTINE INVESTIGATION

Normally the cerebrospinal fluid is clear and colourless. A yellowish tinge of the fluid (xanthochromia) is suggestive of haemorrhage or spinal block.

Coagulum on standing
This occurs in meningitis (tuberculous, syphilitic or septic). Massive clotting takes place in spinal block (Froin's syndrome), due to the great increase in protein.

Presence of blood
If blood is present at the commencement of the flow and later disappears it is often due to the accidental injury of a

blood vessel by the needle. If blood is mixed with the fluid throughout the whole specimen, it is suggestive of haemorrhage into the cerebrospinal space, e.g. subarachnoid haemorrhage.

Cells
The number of cells is counted in a counting chamber under the microscope. The number normally present is 0–5per mm³. In syphilitic conditions the number is from 10–100per mm³. In tuberculous meningitis the number is from 20–400, mainly lymphocytes. In pyogenic meningitis large numbers are present, up to 2 000 or more, mainly polymorphs. The presence of excessive numbers of cells in the cerebrospinal fluid with neighbouring septic conditions (e.g. mastoiditis), indicates the possibility of the onset of septic meningitis.

Bacteria
These are present in meningitis. They are detected by stained film and culture: meningococci in cerebrospinal meningitis; tubercle bacilli in tuberculous meningitis. Other organisms in septic meningitis, e.g. pneumococci, streptococci and H. influenzae.

Chloride
This is normally 120–130mmol/litre (120–130mEq/litre). The chloride is normal in early tuberculous and pyogenic meningitis, only becoming reduced late in the disease.

Glucose
This is normally 2.8–5.0mmol/litre (50–90mg/100ml). It is greatly reduced in meningococcal and septic meningitis. It is less reduced in tuberculous meningitis (under 2.8mmol/litre).

Protein
This is normally 200–400mg/litre (20–40mg/100ml) of cerebrospinal fluid. It is raised in many diseases of the

central nervous system, especially so in tumours and infections of all kinds.

SPECIAL INVESTIGATIONS

Isocitric dehydrogenase
The normal range is the same as for blood, i.e. up to 0.7iu/litre (see also p. 93).

Urea
The percentage of urea in the cerebrospinal fluid is the same as that in the blood (see p. 103).

Tests for syphilis
The VDRL and TPHA (p. 74) are frequently carried out.

Colloidal gold or Lange's test (now seldom performed)
For this test a series of ten tubes are used in which are varying dilutions of cerebrospinal fluid; colloidal gold solution is added. The amount of change occurring is indicated by numbers. Thus 0 for none, 1 for slight change of colour, and 5 for complete precipitation.

In syphilitic diseases of the central nervous system characteristic reactions occur. Abnormal reactions may also be given in multiple sclerosis and encephalitis lethargica, but in these the Wassermann reaction is negative.

Normal fluid	00111000000	
Paretic curve	55555431000	General paralysis of the insane
Luetic curve	00241110000	Tabes dorsalis and cerebrospinal syphilis
Meningitic curve	00001343300	Meningitis (cerebrospinal, tuberculous)

The meningitic curve is not so reliable as an aid to diagnosis as the paretic and luetic curves.

Turbidity
This may be due to pus, blood, or bacteria.

Drug concentration (see Assay of Antibacterial Drugs, p. 231).

	Cells per mm³	Chlorides mmol/litre	Protein g/litre	Glucose mmol/litre	Colloidal gold
Normal	0–4	120–130	0.2–0.4	2.8–5.0	—
General paralysis	10–100	normal	up to 1.0	normal	Paretic curve
Cerebrospinal syphilis	10–100	normal	slightly increased	normal	Luetic curve
Tuberculous meningitis	up to 400	85–110	up to 2.5	0.5–2.8	Meningitic curve
Pyogenic meningitis	up to 2 000	110–120	up to 5.0	0–1.4	Meningitic curve
Tabes dorsalis	0–10	normal	slightly increased	normal	Luetic curve
Multiple sclerosis	0–10	normal	slightly increased	normal	Normal, paretic, meningitic, or luetic curve

Coordination

By coordination is meant the cooperation of certain groups of muscles to carry out certain acts. In diseases of the central nervous system this cooperation is defective, and the patient has incoordination.

Coordination is tested in the following ways:

1. Romberg's sign. The patient stands upright with his feet together and his eyes closed. This is normally possible. If Romberg's sign is positive he sways about and may fall.
2. The patient is instructed to touch his nose with his finger, first with eyes open, and then with the eyes closed.
3. The arms are widespread and the patient is instructed to bring his finger-tips together, first with the eyes open, then with them closed.
4. The patient tries to walk along a straight line.
5. The patient when lying in bed is asked to place one heel on the opposite knee and run it down the front of the leg to the ankle. As in previous tests this is first done with the eyes open, then with them closed.

Incoordination is present in cases of multiple sclerosis, tabes dorsalis, cerebral tumour, and several other diseases of the nervous system.

SPEECH TESTS (see p. 253)

Cranial Nerves

In certain diseases of the central nervous system, e.g. cerebral tumour and other conditions, it is necessary to test the various cranial nerves to see if they are functioning normally.

1ST, OLFACTORY

Small bottles are used containing articles with a powerful smell, e.g. scent, peppermint, etc.

2ND, OPTIC

Part of the optic nerve, the optic disc, can be viewed
directly. Vision can be tested for colour, extent of field
(perimetry) and acuity (refraction tests and test types).
Pupil reflexes (p. 143) also involve the optic nerve.

Eye Tests

OPTIC DISCS

Considerable information can be obtained by the examination of the optic discs through an ophthalmoscope, especially in cases of disease of the central nervous system,
nephritis, etc. The examination is rendered easier by dark-
ness and dilatation of the pupil by homatropine, but this is
not necessary for an experienced observer.

In addition to the optic disc, the retina may also be
examined by an ophthalmoscope and certain disease conditions observed.

COLOUR TESTS

Colour blindness may be tested for by wools of different
colours, by a lamp with various coloured glasses, or by
colour charts, e.g. Ishihara charts.

PERIMETER TESTS

A perimeter is a fixed upright to which is attached a mov-
able curved arm on which objects can be moved to test
lateral vision. In certain ocular diseases and cerebral
tumours the visual fields are considerably diminished. This
is a routine test in cases of cerebral tumour, and the results
are recorded in the form of a circle (Fig. 5/1). The irregular
shaded portion shows average normal vision. The
unshaded central portion shows extent of vision in a particular case, with greatly restricted visual fields due to a
pituitary tumour.

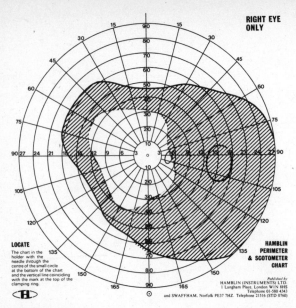

Fig. 5/1   Perimeter test

REFRACTION TESTS

In certain types of eye, vision is defective because the lens
cannot correctly focus an image on the retina. This is corrected by means of glasses. In refraction tests various types
of lens are used until the right one to give correct vision is
found.

TEST TYPES

A common test of vision is that of 'test types'. This consists
of a white card on which are printed black letters of varying
size—a large letter at the top and letters in rows of decreasing sizes underneath. The top large letter should be readable at a distance of 60 metres, the second row at 36 metres,
and so on to the seventh row, which should be readable at 6
metres.

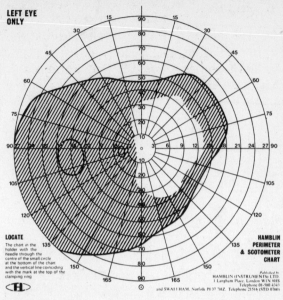

LEFT EYE
ONLY

LOCATE
The chart in the
holder with the
needle through the
centre of the small circle
at the bottom of the chart
and the vertical line coinciding
with the mark at the top of the
clamping ring

HAMBLIN
PERIMETER
& SCOTOMETER
CHART

Published by
HAMBLIN INSTRUMENTS LTD
1 Langham Place, London W1N 8HS
Telephone 01-580 4343
and SWAFFHAM, Norfolk PE37 7HZ. Telephone 21516 (STD 0760)

Fig. 5/1   Perimeter test

The patient is placed at a distance of 6 metres from the card and has to read off as many lines as possible with each eye in turn. The result is expressed thus 6/6, 6/36, 6/60, etc.

6/6. Normal vision.

6/36. Patient can only read at 6 metres what he should read at 36.

6/60. Patient can only read at 6 metres what he should read at 60.

3RD, 4TH AND 6TH, OCULOMOTOR NERVES

These are responsible for the movements of the eyeball. If paralysed, there is defective movement of the eyeball on following the movement of a finger, also a squint and double vision (diplopia) at certain angles. When the 3rd nerve is affected ptosis or drooping of the eyelid is also present.

5TH, TRIGEMINAL

This supplies sensation to the face and also supplies the muscles of mastication. Its function is tested by (1) testing the face for loss of sensation. (2) The patient is asked to clench his teeth while one's hands are held over the muscles of the jaw—any lack of muscular contraction can then be felt.

7TH, FACIAL

This supplies the muscles of the face and if paralysed as in Bell's palsy, there is a distinct difference between the two sides of the face when a muscular movement is attempted, e.g. whistling, shutting the eyes tightly, showing the teeth.

8TH, AUDITORY

This supplies the cochlea (internal ear) and the labyrinth (semicircular canal) which is the organ of balance.

Hearing Tests

AUDIOMETRIC TESTS

Hearing is assessed accurately by an audiometer, an electrical apparatus enabling sounds of varying intensity and pitch to be applied to each ear. The result, expressed on a graph as an audiogram, indicates the degree and type of hearing loss.

WEBER'S TEST

This is a comparison of the bone conduction of the two ears. A tuning-fork is struck, and is placed on the vertex of the skull, and the patient indicates in which ear he hears it louder. In middle-ear deafness it is louder in the affected ear; in nerve deafness it is fainter.

RINNE'S TEST

Test A

A tuning-fork is struck and is held to the external auditory meatus. When the patient ceases to hear it, it is placed on the mastoid process and the patient indicates if he can hear it. Normally he cannot, but in middle-ear deafness he can.

Test B

A tuning-fork is struck and is placed on the mastoid process. When the patient ceases to hear it, it is placed at the external auditory meatus, and the patient indicates if he can hear it. Normally he can, but in middle-ear deafness he cannot. In nerve deafness, provided it is not complete, the result is similar to the normal ear.

AURISCOPY

The eardrum and external auditory meatus can be examined with an electric auriscope or else with an aural speculum, head mirror and lamp. Using either, the auricle (ear) is pulled gently backwards and upwards before inserting the speculum.

LABYRINTHINE (SEMICIRCULAR CANAL) TESTS

Of these the caloric test is most often used. Tap water at 30°C is allowed to flow against the eardrum from an irrigation can 30cm above the patient's head. A stop-watch is used to time the nystagmus (jerking movement of the eyes). It is repeated with water at 44°C. Abnormal responses are seen in Ménière's syndrome and in diseases of the 8th nerve and brain.

9TH, GLOSSOPHARYNGEAL

This supplies the posterior third of the tongue and the mucous membrane of the pharynx. It is tested by (1) taste sensation of posterior part of tongue, e.g. to bitters and (2) tickling the pharynx to see if the reflex is present.

If the 9th nerve is paralysed, other nerves are usually affected.

10TH, VAGUS

This supplies the palate, pharynx, larynx, heart and abdominal contents.

It is tested by (1) noting any deviation of the soft palate, (2) pronunciation of certain words requiring full use of nasopharynx, e.g. tub, egg, etc and (3) paralysis of the larynx is observed through a laryngoscope.

One branch, the recurrent laryngeal, has a course in the upper part of the thorax, and may be paralysed in cases of mediastinal tumour, aneurysm, etc.

11TH, SPINAL ACCESSORY

This supplies some of the muscles acting on the shoulder joint. If paralysed, the patient is unable to shrug the shoulder on the affected side.

This nerve may be damaged in extensive operations on the neck.

12TH, HYPOGLOSSAL

This supplies the muscles of the tongue. The patient is asked to put his tongue out. If the right hypoglossal nerve is paralysed the tongue will be pushed over to the right and vice versa.

This is seen in some cases of hemiplegia.

Tests for Meningeal Irritation

NECK RIGIDITY

With the hand placed behind the patient's head the neck can normally be flexed until the chin touches the sternum.

Flexion of the neck is greatly limited in meningeal irritation.

KERNIG'S SIGN

The patient lies flat on his back on the bed and the thigh is flexed. An attempt is then made to straighten the leg by extending the knee. Normally this can be carried out, but in meningeal irritation the muscles of the thigh pass into a state of contraction and the leg cannot be extended.

The above tests are positive in the majority of cases of meningitis, in subarachnoid haemorrhage and in meningism.

Mental Tests

If an infant is late in sitting up, walking, talking, and gaining control of the bladder and rectum it may or may not indicate mental subnormality, which will be more evident later. Sometimes other indications may be present, e.g. hydrocephalus, mongolism, etc. In some cases a diagnosis of mental subnormality cannot be made definitely until the child is 7 or 8 years old.

DEVELOPMENT SCREENING TESTS (STYCAR AND DENVER)

These detect developmental delay as early in life as possible. The STYCAR (Sheridan Tests for Young Children and Retards) series also test hearing and vision. The Denver tests are designed for use by trained non-medical personnel.

STANFORD-BINET TESTS

These are a series of tests graduated to the age of the individual from the age of 2 years upwards—thus normally—

Child of 3—knows its sex, can name simple everyday objects, etc.

Child of 5—can carry out simple consecutive directions, e.g. put the paper down and close the door, etc.

Child of 7—knows days of week, etc.

GRIFFITHS TESTS

For the age range 0–8 years these tests produce a developmental quotient for the following functions: locomotor, personal-social, hearing and speech, hand-eye coordination, performance and (over 2 years) practical reasoning.

INTELLIGENCE QUOTIENT

This is expressed as the ratio between the real age and the mental age based on a figure of 100. Thus if a child of 10 can only do the tests of a normal child of 5 the IQ is 50 (i.e. $\frac{1}{2}$). If the IQ of a child in its teens is 50–70, it is definitely mentally subnormal, and will probably require continual care and supervision.

MENTAL AGE

This is given by the ability to carry out numerous intelligence tests—thus a child of 14 might have a mental age of 8, i.e. only be able to carry out the tests capable of being done by a normal child of 8.

ADULT MENTAL FUNCTION

Similar tests of mental function (psychometry) can be carried out on adults. Impaired performance may indicate dementia due to physical (organic) disease of the brain, such as tumour or syphilis, or due to severe mental disorder (psychosis).

Records of Electrical Activity

ELECTROENCEPHALOGRAM (EEG)

This is a record of the electrical activity in the brain. It is used sometimes in the location of cerebral tumours and abscesses, and in the investigation of epileptic and other fits.

ELECTROMYOGRAM (EMG)

This is a record of the electrical activity in a muscle, either at rest or during contraction. It is obtained by inserting a needle electrode into the muscle. Different patterns of activity are seen in health and disease.

MUSCULAR ELECTRICAL REACTIONS

A normal muscle will contract on stimulation by an electric current. In cases of paralysis the contraction may be diminished or absent. By testing individual muscles the extent of paralysis can be ascertained, and to some extent the prospect of recovery estimated. The procedure is used in diseases of the nervous system, injuries to nerves, primary muscle disease and to assist in the differentiation of hysterical forms of paralysis.

Reflex Actions

A reflex action is an involuntary response to an external stimulus. The stimulus may be either superficial, e.g. stroking the skin, or deep, e.g. striking a tendon. Changes in the normal response take place in various diseased conditions of the central nervous system, viz the reflex may be absent, exaggerated or altered.

Some of the commoner reflexes will be mentioned.

SUPERFICIAL REFLEXES

Corneal reflex
If the conjunctiva is touched, a reflex closure of the eyelids is produced.

This reflex is used in estimating the degree of anaesthesia or unconsciousness.

Palatal reflex
On touching the soft palate it is elevated. This reflex is often absent in hysterical conditions.

Abdominal reflex
The skin of the abdominal wall is stroked, and this is followed by a contraction of the abdominal muscles.

Plantar reflex
The patient should be lying down with the muscles relaxed. The sole of the foot should be warm. The outer sole is stimulated by pressing firmly with a blunt object, e.g. Yale key or handle of a patellar hammer, and drawing it forward from the heel towards the toes. Normally a slight contraction of the muscles of the leg occurs, and in addition the toes are flexed on the sole of the foot. This is the 'normal flexor response'.

Babinski's sign is present when in the place of the normal flexor response there is an 'extensor response' and the big toe is turned upwards. When this sign is present it indicates definite disease of the central nervous system, involving the upper motor neurones (pyramidal tracts).

In some conditions the reflex may be absent.

DEEP (TENDON) REFLEXES

Knee jerk
If the patient can sit up he should cross one leg over the other. If lying in bed, the knee should be raised, and supported to relax the muscles. The reflex is obtained by striking the patellar tendon just below the patella with a

patellar hammer. In a normal case the leg jerks forward.

In diseased conditions of the central nervous system the reflex may be absent or exaggerated. It is absent in lower motor neurone and sensory nerve disease, e.g. poliomyelitis, neuritis and tabes dorsalis. It is increased in upper motor neurone disease, e.g. hemiplegia and multiple sclerosis.

Tendon reflexes of a similar type are the ankle jerk, the elbow jerk, the biceps jerk and the wrist jerk.

Clonus response

This is the production of a series of contractions in response to a stimulus. The ankle clonus is the commonest example. The knee is bent slightly and is supported by one hand. With the other hand the anterior part of the foot is taken, and suddenly moved upwards, i.e. dorsiflexed; the foot is maintained in this position, and a series of contractions in the muscles in the calf of the leg is produced, causing clonic movements of the ankle.

Patella-clonus is produced with the leg extended, and suddenly pushing down the patella towards the foot. A series of clonic contractions of the muscles of the anterior part of the thigh is produced.

Clonus is only produced in the presence of disease of the central nervous system.

PUPIL REFLEXES

Reaction to light

If a light is flashed in the eye the pupil will contract. A similar reaction is given if the eye is covered and then uncovered.

Reaction to accommodation

The patient is asked to look at a distant object, and then to look immediately at an object held just in front of his nose. Normally the pupil will contract on looking at the nearer object.

Variations in the pupil reflexes take place in diseases of the central nervous system, especially space-occupying lesions in the skull.

Sensation

In many diseases of the nervous system sensation is interfered with, and this can be estimated in various ways.

SENSATION TO TOUCH

The eyes are closed and the patient is tested with a wisp of wool. The contact may not be felt (anaesthesia) or may be felt excessively (hyperaesthesia). The patient may be unable to localise the area touched.

SENSATION TO PAIN

A sharp and blunt object are used, e.g. the point and head of a pin. The patient may not be able to differentiate them. Deep sensation to pain, e.g. by squeezing the muscles of the calf, may be diminished or increased.

SENSATION TO HEAT AND COLD

Small metal containers of hot and cold water are used, and the patient asked to differentiate between them when placed on certain spots. Areas are mapped out on the body where the sensation is abnormal, and the two sides of the body are compared.

DISCRIMINATION, VIBRATION AND POSITION SENSE

Further tests of sensation in seeing if the patient can recognise various objects placed in his hand when the eyes are closed, and if the patient can feel the vibrations of a tuning-fork when placed on the body surface. Position sense may be tested by altering the position of the patient's digit or limb when his eyes are closed, and seeing whether he can describe the altered position.

X-ray Examinations of the Central Nervous System

ANGIOGRAM (p. 222)

ENCEPHALOGRAM (p. 222)

MYELOGRAM (p. 223)

VENTRICULOGRAM (p. 223)

BRAIN SCANS (p. 223)

SECTION SIX
The Urogenital System

The Urogenital System

Collection of Urine

The precautions necessary when collecting a urine specimen depend on the purpose for which it is required. The following types of specimen are collected:

1. Urine for ward or clinic testing. This should be a reasonably fresh specimen collected into a clean container. No special precautions are required unless the patient has a transmissible infection such as typhoid, brucellosis, etc, or is Australia antigen positive when the specimen container should only be handled with protective gloves and tests performed by the laboratory with appropriate precautions (see p. 230).

2. 24-hour urine collection. The bladder is emptied and the urine discarded immediately before commencing the 24-hour collection. During the 24-hour period all urine must be collected including any passed at the time of defaecation. If a specimen is missed the only correct thing to do is to start an entirely new 24-hour collection. At the completion of exactly 24 hours the bladder is emptied, this specimen being included in the 24-hour collection. (Appropriate large containers for the urine collection are available from the laboratory.)

3. Routine laboratory examination of urine. This is usually a mid-stream specimen of urine (MSU) collected as described on p. 153. Precautions required if the patient has a transmissible infection are referred to in (1) above. The specimen should be collected shortly before it is sent to the laboratory accompanied by an inoculated Dipspoon (Medical Wire) or Dipslide (Oxoid) if used.

4. Urine for bacterial counts. The specimen is collected as for (3) but must be sent immediately to the laboratory, accompanied by an inoculated Dipspoon or Dipslide if used.

5. Urine for tubercle bacilli. At least three complete consecutive early morning specimens of urine (EMU) are required (see p. 154) with the precautions for a transmissible infection, as in (1) above.

Ward (or Clinic) Examination of Urine

1. GENERAL APPEARANCE

Note colour, turbidity and presence of blood. Smell is only rarely of value.

2. VOLUME

This may provide vital information concerning fluid balance, e.g. in relation to operations, shock, dehydration, oedema, renal failure, diabetes, steroid therapy, etc.

3. SPECIFIC GRAVITY

This is measured by floating a urinometer in the urine (the calibrations to be checked periodically). This may give information of the kidney's ability to concentrate or dilute urine. (See also p. 156.)

The following tests (4–8) may either be performed separately as described below or else undertaken as a single combined test using Labstix. (See also p. 19 and p. 151.)

4. REACTION (Acidity or Alkalinity)

Universal test papers are very convenient, merely requiring to be dipped into the urine and the colour compared with the colour scale provided. Apart from its intrinsic value, the reaction is also a guide to the type of protein test suitable.

5. TESTS FOR PROTEIN

(a) 25% sulphosalicylic acid, for acid urine. 5ml of urine and 0.5ml of reagent produce a white precipitate if protein is present. If urine is alkaline the boiling test should be used.

(b) Boiling. Add a few drops of acetic acid to the urine in a test-tube and boil. Protein gives a white precipitate.

(c) Albustix or Uristix. The end of the test strip is dipped quickly into the urine and the colour compared with the colour scale. It is a quick test but unsuitable for very alkaline urines, for which the boiling test should be used.

6. TESTS FOR SUGAR

(a) Clinitest is described on p. 28.
(b) Benedict's test is described on p. 28.
(c) Clinistix is a quick preliminary test for glucose only (see p. 28).

7. TESTS FOR KETONES

Acetest and Ketostix will detect both acetone and acetoacetic acid in urine. The tests are described on page 28.

8. TEST FOR BLOOD (Haemastix)

The end of the test strip is dipped briefly into the urine and after 30 seconds compared with the colour chart provided.

9. LABSTIX

This reagent strip tests simultaneously for reaction (pH), protein, glucose, ketones and blood. The test area of the strip is dipped into fresh, clean urine (free from antiseptics, detergents or acid). It is immediately withdrawn and the edge tapped against the side of the container to remove excess urine. The colours of the test areas are then compared with the corresponding colour charts at the times specified, viz immediately, 10 seconds, 15 seconds and 30 seconds. Any abnormal result should be checked by sending the urine to the laboratory.

NB This test does not detect bilirubin (see 10) nor does it detect other sugars such as lactose and galactose. In young children these sugars must be tested for. (See pp. 28, 177.)

10. BILILABSTIX

This test is the same as Labstix (9 above) but also includes a test area for bilirubin.

11. MULTISTIX

This has all the test areas of Bililabstix (10 above) and in addition a test for urobilinogen.

12. TEST FOR PHENYLKETONURIA

Phenistix will detect the presence and concentration of phenylketone (phenylpyruvic acid) in urine. This test was previously performed routinely on all babies but has been replaced by Guthrie's test (p. 96). The test end is dipped into the urine and removed, or moistened against a wet napkin. After half a minute the colour is compared with the chart on the Phenistix bottle. To avoid false negative results the test paper must not be dropped into the urine and left there, nor pressed too firmly or too long against a wet napkin, nor be placed in the napkin while it is on the baby.

Results should be checked by sending a blood specimen to the laboratory for phenylalanine estimation. Any abnormality should be noted on the request form.

In 2–4-week-old infants the urine phenylalanine level should be below 0.5mmol/litre (8mg/100ml).

Routine Laboratory Examination of Urine

In addition to the tests described above, the urine is centrifuged and the deposit examined microscopically. The deposit is composed of the heavier elements such as cells, casts, bacteria and crystals. The deposit may also be cultured to determine the type of bacteria present. Colony counts (see next section) are now becoming a routine procedure. If there is evidence of infection the bacteria are tested for their sensitivity to the different antibiotics.

For this investigation a mid-stream sample of urine (MSU), collected into a sterile container after the urethral orifice has been carefully cleansed, is usually found to be satisfactory in both males and females. The first portion of urine passed should be discarded and only the middle portion collected for sending to the laboratory. Catheterisation has long been considered the only satisfactory method of obtaining a suitable sample of urine (CSU) from females. Catheterisation however carries with it the danger of introducing urinary infection. With care it is usually possible to obtain a suitable non-catheter specimen of urine even from females. This should be routine practice whenever feasible. Catheterisation should be reserved for selected cases where adequate information cannot otherwise be obtained (see white cells, p. 154).

URINE FOR BACTERIAL COUNTS (Colony Counts)

To detect cases of hidden urinary infection, e.g. pyelonephritis, increasing use is being made of bacterial counts. The urine specimen must be transferred to the laboratory immediately or else placed in the refrigerator prior to transfer on the same day. If immediate refrigeration is impracticable, special containers with collection medium can be used (see transport outfits, below). According to Kass, under 10 000 organisms per ml indicates absence of infection; 10 000–100 000 organisms per ml is doubtful; and over 100 000 organisms per ml in three consecutive urine specimens indicates definite infection.

TRANSPORT OUTFITS

In an effort to improve the accuracy and reliability of bacteriological results of urine testing and to eliminate as far as possible the problems created by multiplication of chance organisms while in transit, many laboratories now offer dip inoculum transport outfits, e.g. Dipspoons or

Dipslides. The spoon/slide is dipped into the urine and then returned to its container and transported to the laboratory together with the urine sample. The outfit is incubated overnight and colonies are counted so that an interpretation of any significant growth can be assessed. Counts of over 10^5/ml are usually regarded as significant and counts below 10^4/ml are usually due to contamination.

An alternative transport method is the use of universal containers with boric acid. These are obtainable from the bacteriology laboratory.

URINE FOR TUBERCLE BACILLI

When tuberculous infection of the urinary tract is suspected, at least three complete consecutive early morning specimens of urine should be sent to the laboratory. The urine should be passed in a normal manner into a clean container. The tubercle bacilli are isolated by culture on special media or very rarely by inoculation into guinea-pigs. Normally this takes 4–6 weeks.

Microscopical Examination of Urine

INTERPRETATION OF FINDINGS IN CENTRIFUGE DEPOSIT

White cells
Occasional white cells are normally of no significance. When present in sufficient numbers to suggest infection (viz five or more per highpower field) they are usually reported as 'pus cells'. If in addition to pus cells, a reasonably pure culture of E. coli is isolated, the findings indicate an E. coli urinary infection. Organisms grown from urine in the absence of pus cells are usually contaminants, except in the very debilitated (when catheterisation may be necessary to exclude contamination). A mixed growth of organisms also suggests the possibility of contamination. The finding of pus cells without a causative organism is called 'sterile pyuria'.

It occurs for a short time after any urinary infection has been treated. In nephritis, too, pus cells are seen, usually in small numbers, but casts are also present. Otherwise a sterile pyuria warrants investigation for tuberculosis (see p. 150).

Red cells
The presence of blood in the urine is known as haematuria. It may be due to injury, stones, infection or a growth, affecting any part of the urinary tract. Nephritis is also an important cause of haematuria. A few red cells may be found in normal urine, especially following catheterisation. A non-catheter specimen collected during menstruation may contain red cells as contaminants.

Casts
These are minute structures with parallel sides somewhat resembling elongated sausages. They result from semi-solid material taking on the shape (i.e. forming a cast) of the kidney tubule while passing through. An occasional hyaline (glass-like) cast may be present in the urine of normal people. The number of these hyaline casts increases in states of dehydration, e.g. diabetic coma. In nephritis a number of granular, cellular or hyaline casts are seen, together with a variable number of white cells and often some red cells.

Epithelial cells
These are found in normal urines, usually due to vaginal contamination and also after catheterisation with in-adequate lubricant.

Parasites
These may be found in the urine in certain tropical diseases, e.g. schistosomiasis (bilharzia).

Crystals
Crystals of various salts, e.g. urates and phosphates, are frequently seen and usually reflect the reaction of the urine

and the previous diet, e.g. oxalates following strawberries or rhubarb.

Renal Efficiency Tests

Renal efficiency tests only demonstrate gross disease, and more than half of the kidney substance has to be destroyed before inefficiency is evident. The serum creatinine estimation is now the generally preferred test.

1. BLOOD UREA

If renal function is sufficiently impaired for the blood urea to rise above the normal level of 2.5–7.5mmol/litre (15–45mg/100ml) this can be readily demonstrated.

(a) Laboratory estimation. 2ml of clotted blood is sufficient. (See also p. 103.)

(b) Azostix. A large drop of capillary or venous blood is freely applied over the entire reagent area of the printed side of the strip. After exactly 60 seconds the blood is quickly washed off with a sharp stream of water. Comparison of the colour with the chart provided gives a measure of the blood urea. Any abnormal result is checked by laboratory estimation.

2. WATER DILUTION AND CONCENTRATION TEST

On the first day, the patient, after passing urine, drinks 1 800ml of water within half an hour. Urine is passed at half-hourly intervals for the next 4 hours, and the volume and specific gravity of each specimen is measured. Normally the 1 800ml are excreted within the 4 hours and the specific gravity falls to 1002 or less.

On the second day the fluid intake is limited to 600ml for the 24 hours. Foodstuffs with a high water content should be avoided, e.g. fruit. Urine may be passed whenever the patient desires, each specimen being collected separately, and the volume and specific gravity measured.

Normally the urine does not exceed 900ml for the second 24 hours and the specific gravity reaches at least 1027.

In renal insufficiency the volume on the first day is too little, and on the second day too great, and the specific gravity remains in the region of 1010 for both days.

3. UREA CLEARANCE TEST

There is a great reserve of kidney tissue. Tests of renal function, such as the urea concentration test, indicate extensive kidney damage. The urea clearance test indicates roughly the amount of healthy functioning tissue remaining in the presence of renal disease. The results are read as the percentage of available functioning renal tissue; 80 to 110 per cent is a normal reading. Percentages lower than this indicate damage to the functioning kidneys, decreasing to 10 per cent where the tissue remaining is insufficient, and the patient is in a state of uraemia.

The test is carried out in the following manner.

The patient has a normal breakfast, but without coffee or tea. Between breakfast and the midday meal:

(a) Completely empty the bladder and note the exact time. Discard this specimen.

(b) The patient drinks a glass of water.

(c) A specimen of blood for urea estimation is taken immediately.

(d) One hour after emptying the bladder, empty the bladder again. Label this 'specimen 1' and note the exact time interval on it.

(e) One hour later, take another specimen of urine, label this 'specimen 2' and note the exact time interval on it.

(f) Send the two urine specimens and the blood to the laboratory.

It is important that the bladder be completely emptied on each occasion. The time of collection of the specimens must be accurately measured in minutes, and recorded on the label, e.g. 1st 1 hour and 3 minutes, 2nd 58 minutes.

4. CREATININE CLEARANCE TEST

This is a renal efficiency test. It is more sensitive to impairment of renal function than the blood urea and easier to perform than any of the other renal function tests. All that is required is a 24-hour urine collection and 10ml of clotted blood taken at some time during the 24 hours. It is a measure of the volume of blood cleared of creatinine in 1 minute. Normally this is 70–130ml/minute. It is related to the body area and so the result has to be multiplied by a correction factor for children and fat people. The normal body area is taken to be $1.73m^2$. The patient's body area (a) can be estimated from height and weight tables. The correction factor is then $(\dfrac{a}{1.73})$.

In severe renal failure the creatinine clearance may fall to 5ml/minute.

5. INTRAVENOUS PYELOGRAM (see p. 219)

6. DYE EXCRETION TEST

About 10ml of 0.4% solution of indigo carmine are injected intravenously, and the time observed before the appearance of the dye in the bladder. Normally it should appear in about 5 to 10 minutes, and excretion should be complete in about 12 hours. If the dye does not appear within 20 minutes or excretion is prolonged beyond 15 hours the kidney is inefficient.

The time of appearance may be observed through a cystoscope. (See cystoscopy, p. 159.)

Similar tests may be done with other dyes, e.g. phenol red.

7. PROTEIN SELECTIVITY

This is a test of glomerular damage as in acute nephritis. Two proteins of different molecular size, e.g. transferrin

(MW 90 000) and IgG (MW 160 000) are estimated in serum and urine. The clearance for the larger molecule should be significantly less than for the smaller molecule. If not, the prognosis for recovery by steroid therapy is poor.

CYSTOSCOPY

By means of a cystoscope it is possible to examine the inside of a patient's bladder, use diathermy and biopsy tumour tissue.

The cystoscope consists of a hollow tube, like a small telescope with a light attached. Prior to the examination a sedative is given. The procedure is carried out in the theatre but usually without a general anaesthetic. Local anaesthetic is introduced into the urethra prior to the passage of the cystoscope.

In addition to examining the bladder wall for the presence of tumour or inflammation, cystoscopy enables the ureteric orifices to be seen, and if necessary, ureteric catheters to be introduced. Careful sterilisation of the cystoscope is important.

RENAL BIOPSY

Puncture biopsy allows kidney tissue to be obtained for microscopy without open operation. A preliminary pyelogram establishes the position of the kidneys. The patient lies in the prone position with a sandbag under the abdomen. The bony landmarks are marked out, also the measurements obtained from the pyelogram. The sterile trolley includes sterile towels, swabs, skin cleansing lotions, local anaesthetic, syringe and needles, together with the renal puncture needle (e.g. Franklin-Vim-Silverman or Trucut needle) and a fine exploratory needle. The biopsy specimen is collected into fixative (e.g. neutral formal saline) and sent for histology. The patient is kept in the prone position for 30 minutes to maintain pressure on the kidney and minimise bleeding; and confined to bed for 24 hours, blood pressure and pulse rate being recorded frequently and all urine examined for bloodstaining. Any backache, shoulder pain or dysuria should be reported to the doctor.

Renal biopsy is used to elucidate the nature of kidney disease when the diagnosis cannot be made by the usual methods, provided the patient has two functioning kidneys and there is no bleeding disorder or kidney infection.

LAPAROSCOPY (see p. 32)

Pregnancy Tests

During pregnancy there is a hormone in the blood called human chorionic gonadotrophin (HCG). This passes into the urine and can be detected by the following tests.

1. HAEMAGGLUTINATION INHIBITION TESTS

These include Prepuerin and Pregnosticon. The tests take about 2 hours to perform. Sheep red cells coated with HCG are used and when exposed to rabbit anti-HCG serum are agglutinated. Pregnancy urine prevents this agglutination, its HCG blocking the anti-HCG serum. The tests detect pregnancy about 8 days after the first missed period would have occurred.

2. SLIDE TESTS

These include Gravindex and Prepurex. The tests take about 3 minutes to perform. A drop of the urine is added to a drop of anti-HCG serum. Pregnant urine contains HCG and neutralises the antibody, preventing it from agglutinating latex particles coated with the HCG. The tests detect pregnancy about 37–40 days after the last normal monthly period (LMP).

3. RADIO-IMMUNE ASSAYS

The following sensitive tests are undertaken by the SAS.

(i) Human Chorionic Gonadotrophin (HCG)

An ordinary urine sample is required. It is of value for the following:

(a) Missed abortion, threatened abortion, ectopic pregnancy and early pregnancy. HCG values are lower than usual during pregnancy but above the normal range.

(b) Hydatidiform mole. Assays (including β-HCG) should be done 3 weeks after evacuation of the uterus, then every 2 weeks, until valves are in the normal range, then monthly for 1 year and 3-monthly for the next year.

(c) Choriocarcinoma, other trophoblastic tumours and gonadal teratomas, but see β-HCG (below).

(ii) Beta Subunit Human Chorionic Gonadotrophin (β-HCG)

Serum assays for β-HCG are more sensitive than urine HCG. About 5ml clotted blood suffices for this and AFP. It is of value for:

(a) Detection of hydatidiform mole, choriocarcinoma and monitoring therapy.

(b) Monitoring malignant gonadal teratomas.

These tests are very sensitive and become positive earlier in pregnancy than the older biological tests using mice, rabbits or toads. They can also be used in the detection of hydatidiform mole and chorion epithelioma. Early morning specimens of urine are more concentrated and therefore contain more HCG, but any reasonably fresh specimen of urine is suitable.

Placental and Fetal Monitoring

HUMAN PLACENTAL LACTOGEN (HPL) ASSAY

This is used to monitor the health of the placenta and fetus (and occasionally the growth of certain tumours, e.g. teratomas). 10ml of clotted blood are required. Request forms should include the diagnosis and must state the stage of a pregnancy.

HPL is a peptide normally produced by the placenta (abnormally, by tumours). Its blood level increases most during the first three months of pregnancy when placental growth is greatest and then rises gradually until the 38th week. During the first 6 months, levels lower than normal for the stage of gestation are associated with an increased risk of abortion. Levels less than 4mg/litre after the 34th week indicate serious fetal risk, especially if the level is falling. In diabetes the HPL level is raised and so less than 5mg/litre indicates fetal risk. In cases of Rhesus immunisation levels above the normal range at the 26th week suggests a severely affected fetus.

Serial estimations are of much more value than a single sample. A more commonly used test for monitoring fetal health is urinary oestriol excretion (see below).

OESTRIOL EXCRETION

Estimation of the oestrogen excretion in a 24-hour urine provides an assessment of both placental and fetal function. Oestrogen excretion gradually increases during pregnancy, but before the 28th week the level is so low that its estimation is a lengthy process. After the 28th week more rapid methods of estimation are practicable.

The normal range is very wide, e.g. $35-115\mu$mol/24-hour ($10-33$mg/24-hour) at 36 weeks. A sudden drop in a series of readings provides a clearer guide than a single low reading in reaching a decision to terminate pregnancy.

Exactly timed 24-hour urine is collected into dark Winchester bottles without acid or preservative, initially on two consecutive days and then, if indicated, twice weekly. For non-pregnancy oestrogen excretion, see p. 201.

AMNIOCENTESIS

Amniocentesis may be undertaken from the 14th week of pregnancy until term. It is used for determining the severity of haemolytic disease in the fetus, estimating fetal maturity,

sexing and for detecting whether certain fetal defects may
be present. The technique involves the introduction of a
lumbar puncture needle through the abdominal wall into
the uterine cavity for the removal of liquor amnii.

Before the operation the patient must empty her bladder. Full aseptic precautions are required as to gowns,
masks, etc. The situation of the back of the fetus is determined by palpation. The use of ultrasound minimises the
risk of puncturing the placenta. The skin is cleansed with
weak iodine solution B.P. and anaesthetised with 0.5%
procaine hydrochloride. The needle is then introduced
below the umbilicus of the mother, behind the fetal back. A
20ml syringe is used for extracting the liquor and the fluid
placed in a dark brown bottle. It is immediately sent to the
laboratory, where if it is bloodstained it requires to be
centrifuged and decanted into another dark bottle.

1. *Bilirubin.*
A spectrophotometer is used to study the optical density
deviation produced by the liquor amnii on light
(wavelength 450nm). This gives a guide to the amount of
bilirubin-like substances present. For example, at the 34th
week a deviation of 0.03–1.8 from linearity indicates moderate to severe haemolytic disease.

2. *Assessment of fetal lung maturity*
This is done by estimating the total lecithin level and the
ratio of lecithin to sphingomyelin. Lecithin enables respiratory epithelium to function normally. It acts like a
detergent.

3. *α-Fetoprotein estimation*
This is for detecting open neural tube defects, e.g. spina
bifida, anencephaly or encephalocele. (See also AFP in
blood, p. 81.)

4. *Fetal cells*
These are examined for:
(a) Maturity tests.

(b) Sexing. This is of value for example if Duchenne's muscular dystrophy (affecting males) is suspected.

(c) Chromosome studies (karyotyping) for detecting Down's syndrome (mongolism) and other congenital abnormalities.

If fetal abnormality is suspected, amniocentesis should be performed as early as possible; cell culture for chromosome studies may take upwards of 6 weeks. Abortion after 24 weeks is undesirable and is preferably done before 18–20 weeks (quickening).

TOXAEMIAS OF PREGNANCY

In cases of toxaemia of pregnancy the urine is tested for protein as described on p. 150, and specimens are sent to the laboratory for confirmation and routine examination. In addition, frequent estimation of the blood pressure is carried out, and the fetal heart rate checked.

ASSESSMENT OF FETAL DISTRESS

An abnormal fetal heart rate and meconium staining of the liquor amnii indicate fetal distress. More accurate assessment of the fetal state is provided by:

1. Fetal heart monitoring, using electronic equipment. This records the fetal heart beat in relation to uterine contractions by means of two transducers which are attached to the patient's abdomen.

2. Fetal blood sample examination collected through an amnioscope. This is a slightly conical hollow tube with a light, the narrow end being introduced with aseptic precautions through the vagina and cervix after the membranes have ruptured. Blood is collected from the fetal scalp using a special instrument with a small blade. The blood is collected into heparinised capillary tubing (5cm without bubbles), mixed by drawing a small needle through the tube by a magnet, sealed with gum and sent immediately to the laboratory for estimation of reaction (pH) and blood gases (see p. 100).

TEST FOR PREMATURE RUPTURE OF MEMBRANES

Sometimes the membranes surrounding the fetus rupture before term. If this is suspected a sample of vaginal fluid should be sent to the laboratory in a plain container (universal). Microscopic examination will detect the presence of lanugo hairs or vernix caseosa cells (staining red or orange with 0.05% aqueous Nile blue sulphate). If these are found, a diagnosis of ruptured membranes can be made.

UTERINE SWABS

To take a uterine swab, the patient should be prepared as for a cervical swab (see vaginal discharges, p. 167), but in addition the cervical canal is swabbed clean, and a throat swab passed into the uterine cavity.

Uterine swabs may be taken in cases of puerperal infection and septic abortion. Swabs from the throat of the patient should also be taken to see if she is a carrier of haemolytic streptococci (see p. 118).

STERILITY TESTS

A general medical examination may reveal a cause for sterility in either sex, e.g. endocrine disturbance or debilitating infection. Special investigations are as follows:

Female
1. Pelvic examination to confirm that the reproductive organs are anatomically normal. Abnormalities may be an indication for nuclear sexing (p. 246) or occasionally chromosome study (p. 247).
2. Tests for ovulation. (*a*) Temperature. Take the temperature on each day of the cycle. A rise in temperature in mid-cycle strongly suggests ovulation. (*b*) Blood pro-

gesterone (p. 97). If ovulation has taken place the blood level rises during the luteal phase, viz 20–25th day of cycle, to above 10mg/ml.

3. Tests for patency of Fallopian tubes. (See p. 221, Sterility tests.)

4. Uterine curettings (see below). This may reveal tuberculosis or functional disturbance of the endometrium.

5. Blood progesterone estimation (see p. 97).

Male

1. Examination of the genitalia to confirm that they are anatomically normal.

2. Examination of seminal fluid. Fresh seminal ejaculate collected directly into a clean glass container (never into a condom) is examined in the laboratory for the number of spermatozoa, and also their motility and microscopic structure. Seminal culture, including investigation for tubercle, may be required as part of the infertility investigation or in suspected epididymo-orchitis.

3. Testicular biopsy. A small portion of testis is removed under local anaesthetic, collected into formalin fixative and sent for histology.

Post-coital Test

The wife attends for examination within an hour or two of coitus. She is examined in the left lateral position with the aid of a speculum and an Anglepoise lamp.

1. With a Pasteur pipette a few drops of fluid are taken from the vagina, placed on a slide, covered by a coverslip and examined microscopically for spermatozoa.

2. With a sterile platinum loop a drop of mucus is collected from the cervical canal and similarly prepared for microscopy. If fertility is normal the mucus is penetrated by actively motile spermatozoa. In cervicitis pus cells are seen.

3. A swab for bacteriological culture should also be taken from the cervical canal.

UTERINE CURETTINGS

It is desirable that all curettings from the uterus should be examined microscopically. When there is the possibility of a malignant growth it is essential for this to be done.

The material removed from the uterus should be placed immediately in a small jar or tube containing fixative, preferably Masson's, Bouin's or Susa's fluid, and correctly labelled. This is sent to the laboratory, where it is mounted in wax, and sections cut for microscopical examination.

PAPANICOLAOU SMEAR

This is invaluable in the early diagnosis of cancer. It is also useful for detecting trichomonas infections and other conditions. Its advantage is that it can give the result quickly, and is equally effective in very early cases of cancer.

Cervical Scrape

A speculum is inserted into the vagina with the minimum of lubrication and the cervix is inspected. An Ayre's spatula is applied to the ectocervix. With one side of the spatula blade pivoted in the external os the spatula is rotated to obtain a complete circular sweep over the surface of the cervix. The material on the spatula is spread evenly on a glass slide labelled with the patient's name or number, avoiding too much rotary movement. The smear is immediately fixed while still wet (see p. 244).

Vaginal Smear

Using a special pipette, secretion is obtained from the posterior fornix of the vagina. The secretion is spread *thinly* on a labelled glass slide and immediately fixed while still wet.

VAGINAL DISCHARGES

In cases of vaginal discharge, it is important to discover the organisms present, and for this purpose several different types of specimen may be collected.

In children vulvo-vaginitis may be present, and in this case a vaginal swab is taken.

In adults a vaginal discharge is often associated with Trichomonas vaginalis. This is a protozoon a little larger than a leucocyte. In order to recognise its presence, a drop of discharge is examined on a glass slide, in a fresh, warm condition under the microscope. Alternatively it may be preserved temporarily by using a vaginal swab put in a transport medium which is then transmitted to the laboratory without delay. A specimen taken with a dry swab should be collected at the same time. T. vaginalis can also be detected by Papanicolaou smear (p. 167).

In pregnancy, a vaginal discharge is often due to the presence of thrush caused by a yeast, Monilia albicans, and this can be recognised by examination of a vaginal swab.

Provided the patient is not pregnant a cervical swab should be taken. The vaginal fornices are swabbed dry and a throat swab passed into the cervical canal. If urethral discharge is present a urethral smear and culture should also be collected.

URETHRAL DISCHARGES

In the female the patient should be placed in the lithotomy position, the vulva separated and swabbed down. A finger is then inserted into the vagina, and the urethra 'milked' from behind forward by pressure on the anterior vaginal wall. A sterile mounted loop of platinum wire (sterilised by heating in a flame) is then passed into the urethra, and the material obtained spread thinly on a sterile glass slide, dried without heat, and fixed by adding a few drops of alcohol. Sometimes the material obtained may be transferred to a culture tube.

In the male the urethral orifice is cleaned, and the swab or wire inserted as described. If the discharge is scanty it may be necessary to massage the prostate by a gloved finger in the rectum prior to taking the swab.

Gonococci are frequently found in urethral discharges. Repeated examinations may be necessary to prove or disprove their presence.

The organisms may be cultured by collecting the discharge on a swab. When delay is anticipated a special swab is used and placed in Stuart's transport medium for dispatch to the laboratory (see p. 229).

CHANCRE

At the site of primary syphilitic infection a hard nodule forms. This breaks down to form a shallow ulcer, from the surface of which serous fluid is exuded. This is highly infectious, therefore rubber gloves should be worn when collecting a specimen.

The surface of the sore should be cleaned with a swab soaked in spirit. The sore should be squeezed until serum exudes. A drop is taken with a platinum loop or capillary tube, and diluted with a drop of saline on a slide.

The specimen is sealed with a cover slip, and examined immediately under a microscope, using dark ground illumination for the spirochaetes of syphilis.

FREI TEST

Lymphogranuloma venereum is a venereal disease found in tropical climates. In this country it is sometimes seen in those returning from such areas. The disease is due to a virus and antigen preparations are available from the local public health laboratory. Some of this antigen is injected into the patient intradermally. In a positive case a papule with a necrotic centre appears in about 48 hours.

Chemical Substances in Urine

ADRENALINE AND LIKE SUBSTANCES (see Catecholamines, p. 195)

ALCOHOL

This estimation is carried out in a similar manner to that of blood alcohol (see p. 80).

The figure for urine is usually higher than that given by the blood and is less reliable.

AMINO-ACIDS

Normally relatively small amounts of certain amino-acids (e.g. glycine and glutamine) are present in the urine. Abnormal amounts and types of amino-acid appear in the urine in liver failure and in a number of congenital metabolic diseases.

1. *Total Amino-acid Nitrogen.* Urine normally contains 100–400mg per 24 hours (as estimated by the formol method). This is greatly increased in the conditions mentioned. For this test an exact 24-hours specimen of urine is required, collected into brown bottles containing preservative.

2. *Chromatography.* Three separate specimens of midstream urine are required, each collected into a universal container. Chromatography identifies the individual amino-acids and the approximate amounts of each. Usually 6–10 amino-acids are present, glycine predominating.

3. *Cystine.* A screening test will detect cystinuria, a congenital disorder with excess cystine in the urine. The normal excretion is 0.1–0.4mmol/24-hour.

AMYLASE (see p. 25)

BARBITURATES

About 100ml of urine is usually required. It is a useful screening test for suspected poisoning but blood levels are more satisfactory if available (see Drugs, pp. 87–8).

BENCE-JONES PROTEIN

In the diseases of multiple myeloma and secondary carcinoma of bone, an abnormal protein appears in the urine where it can be detected 2–3 years before blood or bone changes are found. A 24-hour specimen is required.

CALCIUM AND MAGNESIUM

On an average diet 2.5–7.5mmol (100–300mg) of *calcium* are excreted in the urine daily. Nearly three times as much is excreted in the faeces. Excretion is greatly increased on a diet rich in milk and cheese. Diseases causing an increased excretion, e.g. 300–600mg per day, are hyperparathyroidism, hyperthyroidism and multiple myeloma. Urine calcium is low in rickets and defective intestinal absorption. A complete 24-hour specimen of urine is required for the estimation, collected into a container provided by the laboratory. *Magnesium*, normally 7–11mmol/24-hour (168–268mg/24-hour), may be estimated on the same specimen. Renal calculi may be associated with raised calcium or magnesium levels.

CANNABIS

In cannabis intoxication urine levels of cannabis derivatives usually exceed 100μg/litre. About 5ml of freshly collected urine is sent to the laboratory for urgent transmission to the SAS centre for radio-immune assay. Samples more than 24-hours old are not acceptable.

CATECHOLAMINES (see p. 195).

CHLORIDES (see Electrolytes, p. 88)

CREATINE

Normally there is little, if any, creatine in adult urine. Some may be found during menstruation, pregnancy, childhood, athletic activity and starvation. Considerable increase may be found in the muscular disorders, in any condition where there is muscular wasting, following fractures and in hyperthyroidism. A complete 24-hour specimen of urine is required for creatine estimation. It is of some value in assessing the rate of muscle destruction in muscular disorders.

CREATININE

The normal daily excretion of creatinine is about 10mmol (1g) for women and 20mmol (2g) for men. Its excretion is very constant from day to day for a given individual. This constancy provides a check that 24-hour urine collection is complete when a series of such samples is required for chemical or microbiological assay. The creatinine clearance test is described on p. 158.

CYSTINE

The presence of an increased amount of the amino-acid cystine in the urine is characteristic of cystinuria, one of the congenital metabolic diseases. See amino-acids (p. 170).

ELECTROLYTES (Chloride, Sodium and Potassium)

To estimate daily electrolyte excretion a complete 24-hour urine collection is required. Chloride, sodium and potassium may be estimated on the same specimen. The amount of each excreted is normally just sufficient to keep the blood level within normal limits.

Chloride
A normal adult excretes 120–250mmol (7–15g) (expressed as sodium chloride) daily in the urine. This is reduced or absent in salt depletion and also in salt retention with oedema. Depletion occurs in excessive sweating, vomiting or diarrhoea. Retention occurs in renal or cardiac failure and in excessive steroid therapy. For chloride esti-

mation a specimen of urine should be sent to the laboratory. To estimate daily excretion, a complete 24-hour specimen of urine is required.

An appropriate estimate, only to be used when laboratory facilities are not available, is by the method of Fantus: 10 drops of urine are placed in a test-tube; 1 drop of 20% potassium dichromate is added; 2.9% silver nitrate is added drop by drop. The number of drops needed to give a brick-red precipitate gives the number of grams of sodium chloride per litre of urine. The pipette must be washed out with distilled water between each stage. In view of its doubtful reliability this test is almost obsolete.

Sodium

Normally 130–220mmol (3–5g) are excreted daily. This is reduced in sodium retention which is usually associated with chloride retention (see above). In Addison's disease sodium continues to be excreted in spite of a low blood level. This can be controlled by steroid therapy.

Potassium

Excretion varies with diet. Usually it is 25–100mmol (1–4g) daily. In Addison's disease there is diminished excretion in spite of a high blood level. Steroid therapy increases potassium excretion so that the blood level is lowered.

ELECTROPHORESIS

An early morning specimen of urine is usually required. The test is useful for identifying abnormal proteins, e.g. myeloma protein and for FIGLU (see below).

FIGLU (Formimino-glutamic acid) EXCRETION TEST

Excess of this substance appears in the urine of patients with folic acid deficiency when they are given the following test. After fasting overnight 15g of histidine monohydrochloride are given by mouth and washed down with water.

An hour later eating is permitted. Three hours after the histidine the bladder is emptied and the urine discarded. For the following two hours all urine is collected into a bottle containing 1ml of concentrated hydrochloric acid and some thymol crystals. A pre-test specimen of urine is also required for dilution purposes. The FIGLU is detected by electrophoresis, chromatography or using an enzyme method. Normally only small quantities of FIGLU are found. Excess occurs in folic acid deficiency. FIGLU is absent in histidinaemia, a congenital defect in which the enzyme histidase is lacking.

FSH (Follicle Stimulating Hormone) (See Pituitary Gland Investigations, p. 196)

5-HYDROXY-INDOLEACETIC ACID and
5-HYDROXY-TRYPTAMINE (SEROTONIN)

These substances are increased in the urine of many patients with carcinoid tumours. Normal urine contains about 100μg/litre of each. The screening test may detect none or a trace only. Urine is collected as for catecholamine estimation (p. 195).

17-KETOSTEROIDS AND 17-KETOGENIC STEROIDS
(see Urine Tests for Steroids, p. 192)

OESTROGENS (OESTRIOL) (See Oestriol Excretion, p. 162)

PORPHYRINS AND RELATED SUBSTANCES

Porphyrins are formed during the biosynthesis of haemo-globin; 50–250μg are excreted in the urine daily. This amount is too small to be detected by the screening test. Increased excretion occurs in haemolytic anaemias, polycythaemia, liver diseases, fevers and as a result of some drugs and poisons (e.g. lead). There is also a group of diseases with a hereditary factor known as the porphyrias in which there is increased excretion of porphyrins and related substances. Normally a 24-hour urine contains only traces of these viz coproporphyrin <240nmol (<240μg), uroporphyrin <30nmol (<30μg), porphobilinogen (PBG) 45μmol (<2mg) and δ-amino laevulinic acid (ALA) <15μmol (<7mg). Laboratory screening tests will detect excess of the first three. For accurate estimation of porphyrins, etc, a complete 24-hour collection of urine is required, preferably on several successive days. Examination of a single fresh specimen can be of value as a rough guide.

The following points should be noted when investigating suspected porphyria:

1. Tests are negative before puberty in children who will later develop porphyria.
2. Screening tests on urine are negative during the latent phases of intermittent porphyria.
3. Faecal porphyrin estimation should also be done (see p. 38).
4. Positive tests must be confirmed by quantitative analysis and typing of the porphyrins.

PROTEINS

The routine ward tests for protein in urine are given on p. 150. These give a rough guide to the amount of protein in the urine. It is sometimes of value, e.g. in kidney disease, to know approximately how much protein is being lost in the urine daily, as by Esbach's method together with measurement of the daily output of urine.

Esbach's test

An Esbach's albuminometer is used (Fig. 6/1). Urine is added to mark U, followed by Esbach's reagent to mark R. It is stoppered and inverted several times to mix well, and allowed to stand in a vertical position for 24 hours. The amount of protein is then read off directly on the tube

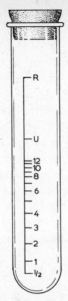

Fig. 6/1   Esbach's albuminometer

calibrations as parts per thousand (i.e. grams per litre). A concentrated urine should be diluted before the test to give a specific gravity of about 1 008–1 010 and the result correspondingly corrected (viz if diluted with an equal volume of water the result should be doubled).

For a more accurate estimation, a complete 24-hour collection of urine should be sent to the laboratory. Other tests for protein are electrophoresis (p. 173) and the test for Bence-Jones protein (p. 171).

REDUCING SUBSTANCES

Tests for reducing substances are described under 'Sugar in urine', p. 28. The nature of a reducing substance is determined in the laboratory by chromatography (see p. 177) and other methods.

STEROIDS (See Urine Tests for Steroids, p. 192)

SUGAR CHROMATOGRAPHY

This is a method of separating and identifying sugars present in the urine. Thus it will distinguish between lactose (associated with lactation) and glucose even if both are present. A fresh early morning specimen is required.

UREA

Urine urea estimation is usually part of a renal function test, e.g. urea clearance test, p. 157. Estimations may occasionally be made on single specimens. A high concentration of urea indicates that the kidney has good concentrating power and is evidence that renal failure is not present. The average concentration of urea over the day is about 2 per cent, and the total daily excretion about 30g. With normal kidney function it is a measure of the breakdown of protein from both food and body.

UROBILIN AND UROBILINOGEN

The bile pigment bilirubin is altered in the intestine to urobilinogen. Some of this is reabsorbed and then excreted by the kidney, the urobilinogen gradually changing into urobilin. The urobilin and urobilinogen in urine, normally 2–5mg/24-hour, are increased in haemolytic jaundice, up to 10mg daily, and reduced in simple obstructive jaundice, usually to less than 0.3mg daily. A fresh sample of urine in a universal container is sufficient for a rough guide (see also p. 19). For accurate estimation a complete 24-hour specimen of urine is collected into a brown bottle containing appropriate preservative, obtainable from the laboratory.

SECTION SEVEN
The Endocrine Glands

The Endocrine Glands

Endocrine glands may secrete too much or too little hormone. Abnormal secretion may be due to a *primary* abnormality in the gland or be *secondary* to an abnormality of the controlling mechanism.

If clinical examination and hormone assay give equivocal results, *dynamic tests* may be used. There are two groups:

1. *Stimulation tests* are used in the diagnosis of inadequate secretion by a gland. The trophic hormone which normally stimulates the gland is administered. A normal response excludes a primary abnormality of the gland; failure to respond confirms it.

2. *Suppression tests* are used in the diagnosis of excessive secretion by a gland. A substance is administered which would suppress a normal gland. A normal response excludes a primary abnormality of the gland; failure to suppress secretion confirms it.

Thyroid Gland Investigations

Thyroid Function Tests (Thyroid Profile)

The following may be estimated on 10ml of clotted blood:
  T_4 (Thyroxine) Estimation
  T_3 (Tri-iodothyronine) Estimation
  T_3 (Tri-iodothyronine) Uptake and/or Thiopac 3
  Free T_4 Index (FT_4I) and Free T_3 Index (FT_3I)
  Thyroid Stimulating Hormone (TSH)

The procedure adopted is along the following lines. T_4 estimation is performed on all samples. If the T_4 is low Thyroid Stimulating Hormone (TSH) assay is performed. If the TSH is high it indicates that the primary failure is in the thyroid, i.e. primary hypothyroidism. If the T_4 is high Thiopac 3 and T_3 measurements are undertaken. From these the FT_3I and FT_4I are calculated. A high level of one or both these indices confirms a diagnosis of hyperthyroidism. If a diagnostic problem still exists after completion of the thyroid profile it should be discussed with the laboratory and further tests may be undertaken, e.g. Radioactive Iodine Test (p. 186).

T_4 (THYROXINE) ESTIMATION

The serum level of thyroxine, the principal thyroid hormone, can be measured by radio-immune assay. It accounts for 90 per cent of the PBI (p. 186), but its estimation is much less affected by outside factors. The results are reported in SI units, the normal range being 55–150nmol/litre (4.5–15μg/100ml or as thyroxine iodine 2–7μg/100ml). It is reduced in hypothyroidism, rising on treatment; and raised in hyperthyroidism, falling on treatment.

T_3 (TRI-IODOTHYRONINE) ESTIMATION

T_3 has four times the biological activity of T_4 but normally the ratio of T_4 to T_3 in blood is 50 to 1. However, in some cases of thyrotoxicosis it is mainly the T_3 that is increased and so its measurement is of practical value. The normal serum T_3 level is 1.3–3.5nmol/litre.

T_3 (TRI-IODOTHYRONINE) UPTAKE AND/OR THIOPAC 3

The test measures the capacity of serum protein to bind T_3. This indicates the number of free sites available to combine with thyroxine. Using Thiopac 3 the results are expressed as a percentage of the standard T_3 uptake, 92–117 per cent being accepted as the normal. It is increased in hypothyroidism (because more sites are unoccupied) and reduced in thyrotoxicosis. It provides a valuable check on T_4 results which can be affected by certain conditions, e.g. pregnancy and the contraceptive pill.

FREE T₄ INDEX (FT₄I) AND FREE T₃ INDEX (FT₃I)

These indices provide a numerical description of the thyroid status. They provide values which are corrected for the serum proteins and are therefore more reliable than serum T_4 and T_3 levels, not being significantly affected by oral contraceptives or pregnancy. The normal FT_4I is 55–145nmol/litre and the FT_3I is 1.4–3.7nmol/litre. One or both indices are increased in thyrotoxicosis and reduced in myxoedema. A similar index used in some hospitals is the Effective Thyroxine Ratio (ETR).

THYROID STIMULATING HORMONE (TSH)

This hormone, produced by the pituitary gland, controls thyroid gland activity. It is estimated by radio-immune assay. The upper limit of the normal range is about 5mU/litre. The level is always increased in untreated primary hypothyroidism, reflecting the pituitary's attempt to stimulate an inadequate thyroid gland into greater activity.

THE TRH (Thyrotrotrophin Releasing Hormone) TEST

TRH is a substance (tripeptide) produced by the hypothalamus which controls the secretion of TSH (Thyroid Stimulating Hormone) by the pituitary gland. After 5ml of clotted blood has been collected for control TSH estimation, $200\mu g$ synthetic TRH in 2ml saline is injected rapidly intravenously. Further blood samples are taken 20 and 60 minutes later for TSH assay.

This test is of value in cases of hyperthyroidism where the serum T_4 and T_3 levels are borderline. The diagnosis of hyperthyroidism is confirmed by finding a rise of less than 2mU above the control level at 20 and 60 minutes. In primary hypothyroidism the basal level is raised and the response to TRH is exaggerated and prolonged. If thyroid failure is secondary to pituitary disease the TSH response is usually absent or impaired. If the cause of the thyroid failure lies in the hypothalamus, the TSH level at 20 minutes may be normal but the 60 minute level is even greater whereas in normal subjects it falls below the 20 minute peak.

RADIOACTIVE IODINE TESTS

1. Urine Excretion Method

After the patient has fasted for at least 2 hours he is given a measured dose of radioactive iodine (^{131}I). Urine is carefully collected into three separate Winchester bottles during the periods: 0–8 hours, 8–24 hours, and 24–48 hours. Alternative methods of collection are used in some hospitals, e.g. a separate container for each specimen passed, noting the time of each collection. The amount of radioactive iodine (^{131}I) excreted is measured by means of a Geiger-Muller counter. In thyrotoxicosis a larger proportion of the iodine than normal is concentrated in the thyroid and so less than normal is excreted in the urine. In myxoedema the reverse occurs.

On the results of the above test, certain cases may be selected for further laboratory tests. A thyroid scan directly measures the uptake of radioactive iodine by the thyroid. The protein-bound radioactive iodine can also be measured.

2. Thyroid Scan

The uptake of radioactive material by different parts of the thyroid gland is mapped out, using a Scintiscan or Gammascan. This distinguishes the overall increase in thyroid activity of Grave's disease from toxic nodular goitre where 'hot' areas are surrounded by cold areas. It is also of limited value in the diagnosis of thyroid cancer.

PROTEIN-BOUND IODINE (PBI)

10ml of clotted blood must be collected into a special container. The average normal PBI is 3–8μg per 100ml. It is reduced in hypothyroidism, rising on treatment; and raised in hyperthyroidism, falling on treatment.

OTHER TESTS OF THYROID FUNCTION

Blood creatine (p. 86) is raised in hyperthyroidism and lowered in myxoedema. Blood cholesterol (p. 84) is raised in myxoedema. The resting pulse rate is raised in hyperthyroidism.

Thyroid Antibodies

Patients with auto-immune thyroiditis produce antibodies against (*a*) their thyroid hormone thyroglobulin, and (*b*) their thyroid tissue itself.

TESTS FOR ANTIBODIES AGAINST THYROGLOBULIN

1. Thyroglobulin Antibody (TA) Test
The patient's serum is tested against latex particles coated with thyroglobulin. Antibody causes the particles to stick together in visible clumps.

2. Thyroglobulin Sensitised Sheep Cells
The serum is tested against sheep cells coated with thyroglobulin. Antibody causes the particles to stick together in visible clumps.

TESTS FOR ANTIBODIES AGAINST THYROID TISSUE

1. Thyroid Precipitin Test
The serum is tested against thyroid tissue extract in agar gel on a slide. The presence of antibody is shown by a line of precipitation in the agar.

2. Thyroid Complement Fixation Test (TCFT)
When antibody combines with thyroid tissue antigen the combination also causes a substance called complement to be fixed to the product. The disappearance of the

complement is then shown by the failure of specially-coated red cells to haemolyse.

3. Immunofluorescent Test for Thyroid Antibody

This test is very sensitive and in some cases is the only way of demonstrating thyroid antibody. The principle of an immunofluorescent test is described on p. 72.

For the above tests 10ml of clotted blood is required. The tests are of value in demonstrating the presence of anti-bodies characteristic of auto-immune thyroid disease. They are also sometimes found in other auto-immune diseases, e.g. pernicious anaemia, and occasionally in healthy people.

Special Signs Associated with Hyperthyroidism (Exophthalmic Goitre)

EXOPHTHALMOS

This is an abnormal protrusion of the eyeball.

VON GRAEFE'S SIGN

The patient is asked to look up and down by following a finger. The movement of the eyelid lags behind the move-ment of the eyeball.

JOFFROY'S SIGN

The patient is asked to depress the head and then look up towards the ceiling with the head in this position. There is an absence of wrinkling of the forehead.

MOEBIUS'S SIGN

On attempting to focus the eyes on a near object, the eyes do not converge.

Parathyroid Gland Investigations

In disturbances of the parathyroid gland the following tests are of value: blood calcium (p. 82), phosphorus (p. 83), alkaline phosphatase (p. 83), parathormone (p. 96), cyclic AMP (p. 87) and urine calcium (p. 171). In hyperparathyroidism the blood parathormone, blood calcium and calcium excretion are increased, also the alkaline phosphatase if the bones are involved, but blood phosphorus is diminished provided there is no kidney failure.

Where the cause for a raised serum calcium is uncertain a cortisone test may be performed. If the calcium level does not fall after 10 days of cortisone treatment it implies that hyperparathyroidism is present. This is because cortisone reduces the gut's sensitivity to vitamin D so that the absorption of calcium is reduced. This lowers the serum calcium in patients not suffering from hyperparathyroidism.

In hypoparathyroidism, sometimes associated with tetany (see below) the blood parathormone, blood calcium and calcium excretion are reduced, blood phosphorus is increased and the alkaline phosphatase is normal. The cyclic AMP rises to peak levels about 20 minutes after injection of parathormone. In pseudohypoparathyroidism it does not.

TETANY

In tetany there is an increased excitability of the nerves and muscles, associated with a low serum calcium and alkalosis.

Chvostek's sign
If the facial nerve is tapped where it crosses the jaw, a spasmodic contraction of that side of the face occurs.

Erb's sign
If a galvanic current is passed, strong muscular contractions are produced.

Trousseau's Sign
Pressure round the circumference of the arm produces tetanic spasm, with flexion at the wrist and metacarpophalangeal joints.

Laboratory Tests
The low serum calcium is characteristic (p. 82). In cases of urgency plasma calcium should be estimated, 5ml of blood being taken into a heparinised container; see also Parathyroid Gland Investigations, p. 189.

Adrenal Gland Investigations

Adrenal Cortex

The adrenal cortex secretes steroids. Their estimation, in blood or in urine, provides an index of cortical function. Blood is easier to collect but indicates cortical activity only at the time of collection. A 24-hour urine reflects the total daily cortical secretion but its accurate collection requires careful supervision (see p. 149). There are also tests to measure the response of the adrenal cortex to stimulation (ACTH) and suppression (dexamethasone). See also ACTH under *pituitary*.

BLOOD TESTS FOR STEROIDS

1. Plasma 'Cortisol' (11-HydroxyCorticoSteroids, 11-OHCS)
'Cortisol', as measured by fluorimetry, includes corticosterone but is mainly cortisol. The normal level is 150–600nmol/litre (6–22μg/100ml) in adults. It varies considerably during the day, with a minimum just after midnight and a maximum at about 08.00h. It opposes the effect of insulin in the control of carbohydrate metabolism. Plasma 'cortisol' is raised in adrenal overactivity whether

primary (Cushing's syndrome) due to hyperplasia, adenoma or carcinoma of the adrenal cortex or secondary (Cushing's disease, see ACTH). Other causes of raised 'cortisol' include pregnancy, contraceptive steroids and oestrogen treatment of prostatic carcinoma. Certain drugs, e.g. mepacrine and spironolactone, give falsely high levels. For patients on drugs see Other Specific Steroids, below.

The patient need not be fasted, but all forms of stress must be avoided before collection of 5ml of blood into a heparin tube between 08.00 and 10.00h (or, when investigating circadian rhythm, between 22.00 and 24.00h).

2. Aldosterone

Aldosterone promotes potassium excretion and sodium retention. It is estimated in patients with hypertension who have a low plasma potassium. The aldosterone level is affected by diuretics, such as thiazides, frusemide and spironolactone, purgatives, liquorice derivatives, e.g. carbenoxolone, and oral contraceptives. All such drugs should be stopped for at least three weeks before aldosterone assay. The patient must also receive adequate sodium (>100mmol/24-hour) and potassium (50–70mmol/24-hour) as an inpatient for at least 3 days. Aldosterone assay should only be done if the plasma potassium is less than 3.7mmol/litre. 10ml of blood is collected into a heparin tube early in the morning before the patient has even raised his head off the pillow.

In aldosteronism the plasma aldosterone exceeds 300mmol/litre. In primary aldosteronism due to a tumour (Conn's syndrome) the plasma renin is low. In aldosteronism which is secondary, e.g. to a renal lesion, the plasma renin is high. Renin estimation can be performed on the same sample of blood when indicated by a high aldosterone level.

3. Other Specific Steroids

Other individual steroids may be measured by special techniques (radio-immune assay or competitive protein binding). These enable cortisol to be measured in patients on drugs such as mepacrine or spironolactone which interfere with the simpler fluorimetric method. Other steroids measured in this way include 17-hydroxyprogesterone, raised in congenital adrenal hyperplasia (see also urine pregnanetriol) and 11-deoxycortisol, raised in adreno-cortical insufficiency.

URINE TESTS FOR STEROIDS

1. Free Cortisol

Most of the plasma cortisol is bound to protein but only the free cortisol is physiologically active. This is also the only part of the cortisol which is filtered out into the urine. So if properly collected, with complete absence of stress on the day preceding and on the day of the test, it provides a good assessment of active cortisol. The normal 24-hour excretion is <400nmol (180μg). Increased levels have the same significance as raised plasma 'cortisol' but provide a more sensitive index of adreno-cortical overactivity.

2. Total 17-OxoGenic Steroids (T-17OGS, also called 17-HydroxyCorticoSteroids or 17-OHCS, previously known as 17-Ketogenic Steroids)

This group includes cortisol and closely related compounds. The normal 24-hour excretion is 17–70μmol (5–23mg). Raised levels have the same significance as for free cortisol (above) and plasma 'cortisol'.

3. 17-Oxosteroids (17-OS, previously 17-Ketosteroids)

These measure the products of androgens and closely related substances. The 24-hour excretion in females is 10–70μmol (5–18mg) and is almost entirely from the adrenal cortex. In males it is 20–100μmol (8–25mg) of which 10–20 per cent is derived from the testis as products of testosterone. There is a non-specific reduction of 17-OS excretion in many illnesses. High levels occur in some forms of virilism.

4. Pregnanetriol

Estimations are of value in the investigation of congenital adrenal hyperplasia (see also Oxygenation Index below) and disorders of ovulation, and in monitoring therapy. The normal excretion is:

	μmol/24hours
Children	0–4.8
Women:	
Follicular phase	0.3–5.3
Luteal phase	2.7–6.5
Men	1.2–7.5

For initial investigation the patient must not be on cortisol or any synthetic analogue. No special preparation is required. Send complete 24-hour urine to laboratory for addition of 10ml of 2% boric before onward transmission of 25ml aliquot to SAS.

5. 11-Oxygenation Index

This relatively simple test is of great value in diagnosing congenital adrenal hyperplasia. It can be performed on any sample of urine. A 24-hour collection is unnecessary unless pregnanetriol (above) is being assayed at the same time. Normally the index is less than 0.5. This value is exceeded in various forms of congenital adrenal hyperplasia. The test is unreliable during the first week of life and in severe diarrhoea. Treatment with cortisol or cortisone gives a normal index but prednisone or prednisolone can elevate it.

STEROID EXCRETION TEST

This is no longer considered a sufficiently sensitive test of adrenal cortical function. It has been replaced by the Synacthen or ACTH (stimulation) test which detects adrenal cortical insufficiency (Addison's disease). Overaction of the adrenal cortex is detected by the Dexamethasone Suppression test.

SYNACTHEN (ACTH) TEST

The substance measured in this test is the plasma cortisol.

Screening Test

At 09.00h 2ml of blood are collected into a heparin tube and sent immediately to the laboratory. An intramuscular injection of 250µg Synacthen in 1–2ml of normal saline is then given. At 09.30h a further 2ml sample of blood is collected into a heparin tube and again sent immediately to the laboratory.

The plasma cortisol in the 09.00h specimen should be 0.2–0.7µmol/litre (8–26µg/100ml). At 09.30h the plasma cortisol should be increased by at least 0.2µmol/litre (7µg/100ml) to reach a minimum level of 0.5µmol/litre (18µg/100ml). Lesser values indicate Addison's disease.

Definitive Test

At 09.00h 2ml of heparinised blood are collected as before. Over the next 5 hours an intravenous infusion of 0.5mg Synacthen in 500ml of normal saline or 5% dextrose is given at the rate of approximately 0.1mg Synacthen per hour. During the procedure a 2ml heparinised sample is collected every hour. Each sample is sent immediately to the laboratory for separation of the plasma. The plasma cortisol should reach 0.8–1.4µmol/litre (30–50µg/100ml) in at least one sample. Failure to reach this level indicates Addison's disease.

DEXAMETHASONE SUPPRESSION TEST

A complete 24-hour urine collection is made on five successive days. That from day 1 is the control. On days 2 and 3, dexamethasone 0.5mg is given orally every 6 hours (i.e. eight doses). On days 4 and 5, dexamethasone 2.0mg is given orally every 6 hours (i.e. another eight doses).

The substance measured in this test is the urinary 17-hydroxy-corticosteroid. Normally the level on the control day is 8–33μmol/day (3–12mg/day). After the 0.5mg doses the level falls to less than 7μmol/day (2.5mg/day) and after the 2mg doses none can be detected.

In Cushing's syndrome due to overactivity of the adrenal cortex from hyperplasia the 17-hydroxycorticosteroid excretion is increased to 33–100μmol/day (12–36mg/day). Oral dexamethasone produces a reduction in the amount excreted, indicating that the overactive cortex can still respond in the same way as a normal gland.

In Cushing's syndrome due to tumour of the adrenal cortex the urinary excretion is increased to 50–160μmol/day (19–60mg/day) and there is no reduction following oral dexamethasone.

OTHER TESTS FOR DISEASES OF THE ADRENAL CORTEX

Blood pressure (p. 107).
Electrolytes in blood (p. 88), and urine (p. 172).

Adrenal Medulla

CATECHOLAMINES IN URINE

Some cases of high blood pressure are due to an adrenal medullary tumour (phaeochromocytoma) which secretes excessive adrenaline or noradrenaline into the blood. There is consequently an excess of adrenaline breakdown products in the urine, in the form of catecholamines, including VMA (Vanil Mandelic Acid). Excess catecholamine excretion also occurs with a neuroblastoma, a childhood tumour of the sympathetic nervous system. Normally less than 150 micrograms are excreted per day. For their estimation a complete 24-hour specimen of urine must be collected in a clean Winchester bottle containing 20ml of concentrated hydrocholoric acid. The bottle must be well sealed and sent to a laboratory prepared to undertake the test.

NB For at least 48 hours prior to the test the patient must not eat food containing vanilla, e.g. tomatoes, bananas, cakes, sweets, coffee or tea. Aldomet should not be given for at least a week before the test. Any drugs taken should be noted on the request form.

Pituitary Gland Investigations

PERIMETER TESTS

Perimeter tests (p. 133) may show evidence of pressure on the optic nerve by a tumour in the region of the pituitary gland.

X-RAY

X-ray of the pituitary fossa may show enlargement by a tumour. X-ray also helps to show bone changes in acromegaly.

Anterior Pituitary Hormones

The anterior pituitary produces a number of trophic hormones which control the function of other glands. A pituitary tumour may secrete hormone, e.g. prolactin produced by a prolactinoma. A pituitary tumour is also one of the causes of damage to the pituitary gland, resulting in a reduction in the blood level of other pituitary hormones, generally in the following order: MSH (Melanocyte Stimulating Hormone), the gonadotrophins FSH (Follicle Stimulating Hormone) and LH (Luteinising Hormone), GH (Growth Hormone), TSH (Thyroid Stimulating Hormone) and finally ACTH (Adrenocorticotrophic Hormone). It is now possible to measure the blood levels of these hormones, usually by radio-immune assay. The laboratory should be consulted if an assay is required.

ASSESSMENT OF ANTERIOR PITUITARY FUNCTION

Pituitary function may be assessed by estimating the blood level of trophic hormones and measuring their response to dynamic tests such as the Insulin Tolerance Test (ITT), the Glucagon Test, the Clomiphene Test, the Luteinising Hormone and Follicle Stimulating Releasing Hormone (LRH) Test and the Combined Test of Anterior Pituitary Function.

Prolactin
Serum prolactin assay is of value in the investigation of pituitary/hypothalamic disease, galactorrhoea, infertility and gonadal disorders. 5ml clotted blood is collected between 09.00 and 11.00h, early in the week, avoiding any stress which causes prolactin levels to rise. Most disorders of its secretion result in raised serum prolactin levels, including prolactinoma, the commonest hormone-secreting pituitary tumour. Low serum prolactin is rare but can occur after severe postpartum haemorrhage from pituitary infarction, preventing breast feeding.

Adrenocorticotrophic Hormone (ACTH)
ACTH stimulates the adrenal cortex to produce cortisol. The normal plasma ACTH level varies from 8–50ng/litre at 09.00h to 1–17ng/litre at 20.00h. Usually blood is collected between 09.00 and 10.00h. It is essential to use a plastic (not glass) syringe. 15ml is taken into an ice-cooled heparin tube and sent immediately to the forewarned laboratory. Its assay distinguishes between primary and secondary adrenal insufficiency, plasma ACTH being raised in the former and reduced in the latter. It also assists in determining the cause of Cushing's syndrome once this has been diagnosed. In adrenal adenoma and carcinoma ACTH is undetectable. High normal or slightly raised

levels suggest adrenal hyperplasia due to excess pituitary ACTH (Cushing's disease). Values above 200ng/litre suggest ectopic ACTH from a hormone-secreting tumour of lung or other site.

(Human) Growth Hormone (HGH or GH)

Secretion of growth hormone is very irregular. The normal serum level is 0–50mU/litre (0–7.7ng/ml) but can vary greatly over a few minutes. So results can be misleading unless there is a gross increase as in acromegaly and gigantism. The CSF level is always below 5mU/litre even with an HGH-secreting tumour unless it has extended outside the sella turcica when higher values occur. HGH deficiency is demonstrated by the Insulin Intolerance Test.

Insulin Tolerance Test (ITT)

This is also called the Insulin Stress Test or Insulin Induced Hypoglycaemia Stimulation Test. It is used in the investigation of hypopituitarism and provides information about the secretion of growth hormone (HGH) and adrenocorticotrophin (ACTH, assessed from 'cortisol' levels). It should be performed under constant medical supervision with 40–50% glucose solution ready for intravenous injection in case of severe hypoglycaemia. The patient has to fast overnight and details of the test are available from the laboratory. It is contra-indicated in heart disease and epilepsy (see glucagon test, below). Most normal subjects reach an HGH level of at least 30mU/litre during the test. Undetectable HGH indicates total HGH deficiency and below 15mU/litre partial HGH deficiency. With such low figures blood glucose levels must be checked to ensure that hypoglycaemia actually occurred.

Glucagon Test

This test can be used for the detection of hypopituitarism in children or in patients with heart disease or epilepsy. Glucagon is given as a single dose of 0.5mg in children, 1.0mg in adults under 90kg and 1.5 for those over 90kg.

Blood samples are taken for growth hormone (HGH) and 'cortisol' at 0, 60, 90, 120, 150, 180, 210 and 240 minutes. In normal subjects serum HGH levels usually start to increase by 90 minutes and rise to above 20mU/litre.

Clomiphene and Gonadotrophin Releasing Hormone (LH/FSH-RH) Tests

These tests for pituitary gonadotrophin secretion are of limited diagnostic value. They are of no value if serum LH and/or FSH values are high, indicating primary gonadal failure. They can be of assistance in assessing the amount of pituitary tissue present after attempted pituitary ablation. Details are available from the laboratory.

Combined Test of Anterior Pituitary Function

This test provides an assessment of ACTH, HGH, TSH, prolactin and gonadotrophin secretion. The patient fasts overnight. An intravenous cannula or butterfly needle is inserted into an antecubital or forearm vein. By injecting 2ml of saline-heparin (20ml saline with 1 000 units heparin) from time to time the system is kept patent. After allowing 45 minutes for the patient to relax, basal samples of blood are collected for glucose, HGH, TSH, prolactin, FSH and LH. At zero time soluble insulin (measured in a tuberculin syringe) is injected followed by $200\mu g$ TRH and $100\mu g$ LH/FSH-RH in 5ml sterile water intravenously and washed in with 2ml of saline-heparin. The amount of insulin injected depends on the clinical state. If hypopituitarism is definitely suspected 0.1 units per kg body-weight is given. If suspicion is less certain, as with delayed puberty, the standard dose of 0.15 units/kg is given. Where insulin resistance is suspected, as in acromegaly or Cushing's syndrome 0.2–0.3 units per kg is used. To be effective blood glucose should fall to 2.2mmol/litre (40mg/dl) or less and be at least half the basal level. Slight sweating and faintness should occur but 40–50% glucose solution should be ready for injection in case of severe hypoglycaemia, with constant medical supervision.

Normally the basal 'cortisol' is at least 140–170nmol/litre (5–6µg/100ml) and rises to 500nmol/litre (18µg/100ml). The increase above basal level should be at least 195nmol/litre (7µg/100ml). Deficient rise in cortisol indicates deficient ACTH secretion provided the adrenal glands are responsive, demonstrable by the Synacthen test. HGH response is as described under the Insulin Tolerance Test and TSH response as for the TRH (Thyrotrophin Releasing Hormone) test.

EFFECTS OF THE ANTERIOR PITUITARY ON OTHER ENDOCRINE GLANDS

In Simmond's disease (hypopituitarism) there is often insufficient thyrotrophic hormone to stimulate the thyroid adequately. So thyroid function tests may show the changes of hypothyroidism, but serum TSH is reduced whereas in primary hypothyroidism it is increased (p. 185). Similarly there may be insufficient ACTH to stimulate the adrenal cortex adequately. So tests for adrenal cortical activity often show similar results to Addison's disease. However, the Synacthen test (p. 194) differentiates them, giving a normal response in Simmond's disease, unlike Addison's disease.

In Cushing's disease due to basophil adenoma of the pituitary, too much ACTH is produced, stimulating the adrenal cortex excessively. So the tests will show evidence of excessive adrenal cortical function. The Dexamethasone Suppression Test distinguishes this from primary adrenal overactivity (Cushing's syndrome). In addition plasma ACTH can now be estimated. This is a costly procedure and the laboratory should be consulted.

Assessment of Posterior Pituitary Function

The main effect of lesions of the posterior pituitary is a reduced secretion of Antidiuretic Hormone (ADH) and so the patient tends to develop diabetes insipidus, character-ised by the passage of a large volume of dilute urine. The following tests enable the diagnosis to be confirmed and the severity of the condition to be assessed.

1. WATER DEPRIVATION TEST

The patient is totally deprived of fluid for several hours so that his body-weight falls by about 3 per cent. Urine is collected at about hourly intervals. Normally the urine specific gravity increases to well above 1020. If ADH is deficient it does not rise above 1010. For the small volumes of urine involved it is more practicable to have the osmo-lality measured by the laboratory. Normally this rises to 800mosm/kg or more but in diabetes insipidus it fails to do so. Conversely the plasma osmolality, measured from blood taken into a heparin tube normally does not rise above 300mosm/kg. In diabetes insipidus it exceeds this figure, the blood becoming more concentrated as a result of dehydration.

2. ADH STIMULATION TEST

This is only necessary if the water deprivation test results indicated diabetes insipidus. The patient is given as much fluid as he wishes. 20µg des-amino, d-arginine vasopressin (DDAVP) is instilled intranasally. Over the next 4 hours urine is collected hourly. In patients with cranial diabetes mellitus the urine osmolality rises to 600mosm/kg or more. Failure to respond suggests that the dilute urine is due to kidney disease, i.e. nephrogenic diabetes insipidus.

Gonadal Endocrine Function Investigations

TOTAL NON-PREGNANCY OESTROGENS

Complete 24-hour urine specimens are required. The normal ranges are as follows:

	nmol/24 hours
Children under 10 years	0–80
Women:	
Follicular phase	20–150
Mid-cycle peak	60–300
Luteal phase	45–290
Post-menopausal	10–55
Men	5–40

Multiple assays are needed to detect ovulation. Excretion is increased in precocious puberty and gynaecomastia. It is reduced in amenorrhoea due to hypogonadism. In primary hypogonadism serum FSH values are high but in the secondary form they are low. Cyclical FSH and LH changes may be seen in precocious puberty. For oestrogen excretion in pregnancy, see p. 162.

OESTRADIOL-17β

This provides an assessment of ovarian function similar to the total non-pregnancy oestrogens. It can be estimated from a 24-hour urine and from a 5ml heparinised sample of blood. Several samples at weekly intervals are recommended for assessment of ovarian activity, e.g. in dysfunctional uterine haemorrhage. High levels occur with oestrogen-secreting tumours which can arise in ovary, testis and adrenal glands.

PROGESTERONE

Serum progesterone assay provides evidence of luteal function. It is of value in the treatment of infertility but should only be undertaken after consultation with the appropriate SAS centre. Levels of 0.3–2nmol/litre are normally present during the proliferative phase, rising during the luteal phases to a peak value of up to 60nmol/litre by about the 24th day of the cycle. 10ml of heparinised blood are required.

TESTOSTERONE

The normal plasma testosterone level is 10–20nmol/litre (280–$600\mu g/100ml$) in males and 1–2.5nmol/litre (27–$70\mu g/100ml$) in females. It is increased in women with virilising tumours, in XYY males and in boys with precocious puberty. Male testosterone levels in a patient with a female appearance characterises the testicular feminisation syndrome. Decreased levels occur in hypogonadism (including Klinefelter's syndrome), hypopituitarism, undescended testes and post-traumatic impotence. 5ml of blood in a heparin tube are required.

SECTION EIGHT
X-ray Examinations

X-ray Examinations

It is not proposed to enter into detailed descriptions of these procedures, but x-ray examinations are carried out on so many patients that it is well to have a rough idea as to their nature and the preparation which may be necessary.

X-rays are invisible to the human eye but have the ability of exciting a fluorescent screen or acting on a photographic emulsion to produce a visible image on the screen or a permanent record on an x-ray film, the radiograph. Fluoroscopic screening enables organs to be visualised directly. This is chiefly of value for examining movements such as the act of swallowing, and the peristalsis of the stomach.

X-rays can penetrate matter, and the penetration depends on the thickness and density of the parts examined. Thus bones will appear as dense opaque structures, soft tissues will be more transparent and air contained in the lungs or abdomen will be completely transparent.

Opaque materials can be introduced into various organs to make their outlines clearly visible on screen or radiograph. Barium sulphate emulsions taken by mouth or administered as an enema are used to opacify the alimentary tract. Iodine-containing solutions injected intravenously will be excreted in the urine to outline the renal tracts. Similar solutions can be injected directly into veins, arteries or by catheter into the heart to demonstrate the anatomy and functional state. A recent advance has been the injection of various radio-isotopes, e.g. technetium, which enables organs such as the brain, bones, liver and spleen to be defined by scanning. By means of a special computer even whole body scanning is becoming possible. Modern apparatus is designed to reduce radiation to the patient while increasing the clarity of the image. Television is now used to intensify screen examinations. Nevertheless x-rays do have harmful biological effects and excessive use should be avoided.

Ultrasound is an alternative to x-rays which avoids the use of ionising irradiation. High frequency sound waves which are inaudible to the human ear can penetrate tissue and outline internal organs. An image is produced on a TV screen and recorded on Polaroid film. Liver, gall bladder, spleen, kidneys, uterus and ovaries are much more clearly demonstrated by ultrasound than by straight x-ray.

Alimentary System

A plain radiograph of the abdomen can be most informative, particularly in the investigation of the 'acute abdomen'. The soft tissue shadows of liver, spleen and kidneys can often be identified and their size assessed. Pathological calcifications due to calculi (stones, pp. 211 and 219), glandular calcification or vascular calcification are shown. Distension of gut shadows with fluid levels will indicate intestinal obstruction and establish whether it involves small or large gut. Air below the diaphragm signifies a perforation of the gut.

Ultrasound examination will decide whether an abdominal mass is solid or fluid-containing, and is of value in demonstrating aneurysms.

BARIUM SWALLOW

This is a modified barium meal (see below), and is used when it is expected that a lesion of the oesophagus is present. The patient is prepared as for a barium meal, but swallows a smaller amount of a more concentrated emulsion, and its course is watched under the fluoroscopic screen from the moment of entering the mouth.

Obstruction of the flow may be due to a stricture, a growth, or, at the lower end, to the condition known as achalasia of the cardia.

If some external mass is pressing on the oesophagus, e.g. mediastinal growth, aneurysm, the course of the oesophagus will be distorted, and obstruction may be present.

A diverticulum of the oesophagus becomes visible as a barium-filled pouch. A hiatus hernia can also be demonstrated.

Examination of the oesophagus is carried out as the first part of a routine barium meal.

BARIUM MEAL

The night prior to the examination the patient is given an aperient if constipation is present. Nothing is given by mouth from the evening before the barium meal.

In the x-ray department, the patient stands behind an x-ray screen and swallows about 300ml of an emulsion containing barium sulphate. The filling of the stomach is observed, and films are taken at the time and at various intervals during the next 20 minutes. A *follow-through examination* may be requested at the same time (p. 210).

Double contrast radiography is a technique for detecting small alterations in the gastric mucosa which may be invisible by ordinary barium meal. It involves the introduction of gas into the stomach (usually from special gas tablets) as well as barium. This provides a double outline which enables small lesions such as early gastric cancer to be seen.

Stomach

If a gastric ulcer is present a crater may be seen which will fill with barium, and the small quantity of barium in this crater may be observed some hours after the stomach has emptied of the main mass.

If the ulcer is long-standing, the stomach may be of an 'hourglass' shape, due to scarring and contraction.

If a growth is present the stomach outline is often irregular and ill-defined. It may show a filling defect. In early gastric cancer the mucosal folds show an altered pattern.

Pyloric stenosis may be present, leading to dilatation of the stomach, and considerable delay in emptying—this may be due either to an ulcer or a carcinoma. The normal time of emptying is about 4 to 5 hours for a barium meal.

If a gastro-enterostomy has been performed previously, a barium meal will demonstrate whether it is working satisfactorily.

Duodenum

The first part of the duodenal shadow forms a 'cap' which is often irregular in cases of duodenal ulcer. A crater may be seen, or a duodenal ulcer may cause pyloric stenosis. Adhesions of a diseased gall bladder may cause irregularity of the duodenal outline. Diverticula of the duodenum may be demonstrated.

'FOLLOW-THROUGH' EXAMINATION

This is a more prolonged method of examination after a barium meal, in which further radiographs are taken during the next 3–6 hours or so, and the course of the barium through the intestinal tract is followed.

Small Intestine

In Crohn's disease the barium may show a narrowing of the ileum known as the 'string sign'.

Large Intestine

The outline of the bowel may show a constant filling defect due to a growth. Diverticula may be seen in cases of diverticulosis. In Hirschsprung's disease the enormously distended colon may be demonstrated. Barium enema however provides a much better method of examining the colon.

BARIUM ENEMA

The preparation requires an emptying of the bowel to allow free passage of the injection. The methods used vary between hospitals. A satisfactory regimen is to give a gentle laxative, e.g. Dulcolax tabs 2 nocte on three successive evenings, starting four days before the barium enema. On the day before the barium enema fluids only are given and on the morning before the examination a phosphate disposable enema or a suppository is given. In the morning a light breakfast is allowed. The patient is taken to the x-ray department where an enema of 900–1200ml of an emulsion of barium sulphate is administered.

The filling of the bowel is watched on the screen, and radiographs of the completed results are taken. The double contrast technique, involving the introduction of gas as well as barium, is now being used with increasing frequency. It enables small mucosal lesions to be detected which might otherwise be missed.

Barium enema is used to demonstrate obstructions due to malignant growths, the presence of diverticulosis, strictures, and the great dilation found in Hirschsprung's disease. In chronic ulcerative colitis the outline of the bowel has fine irregularities. If no obstruction is present, the enema will pass as far as the caecum.

GALL BLADDER

A straight radiograph of the gall bladder may demonstrate the presence of stones, but only 10 per cent of gall stones are opaque to x-rays.

Cholecystography
This is a much more satisfactory method of examination. It consists of giving the patient an opaque medium which is excreted by the liver and concentrated in the normal gall bladder. If the gall bladder fills with the medium, it is rendered opaque to x-rays. The procedure, which should only be undertaken on patients who are not jaundiced, is as follows:

A light meal free from fat—e.g. dry toast and tea—is given at 17.00h, and at 18.00h the patient is given the medium in the form of tablets, followed by a drink of water to remove the taste. The patient then goes to bed, and no food or drink except water (at least three glasses) are allowed. At 09.00h the following morning, a radiograph of the gall bladder region is taken. A meal containing fat is then given, and a further radiograph taken half an hour later.

If the gall bladder is normal, it is shown filled with medium, and empties after the fat meal. If the gall bladder is diseased, it is unable to concentrate the medium, and will not show.

This is a rough guide, but many different conditions may exist. Sometimes the medium will outline the gall bladder, and demonstrate stones which were not visible on a straight x-ray.

The fact that the medium has not concentrated in the gall bladder may rarely be due to other factors besides the gall bladder itself.

Intravenous Cholangiogram

Another opaque medium, e.g. Biligrafin can be injected intravenously, or infused over one hour to outline the bile ducts. Films are taken at 30, 60 and 90 minutes after injection. This may demonstrate bile duct obstruction, e.g. from a growth or stone. It is of no value in jaundiced patients.

Percutaneous (Transhepatic) Cholangiogram

This involves direct injection of contrast medium into the biliary tree for the investigation of obstructive jaundice. Bleeding, clotting, prothrombin times and platelet count are first determined in order to exclude any bleeding tendency. Antibiotic cover is given for 24 hours before the test. The patient is sedated, e.g. by Valium 10mg one hour before the examination. Metal markers are attached to the skin of the epigastrium and right side. A plain x-ray is taken to check the liver size, position and relationship to the metal markers. Then with full aseptic precautions a long thin needle is introduced between the lower right ribs in the lateral line. The progress of the needle is watched under fluoroscopy. As soon as the lumen of the bile duct is reached, contrast medium enters it, outlining the biliary tree. It enables obstruction from stone, stenosis or carcinoma to be demonstrated. After the investigation the patient is kept in bed for 12–18 hours and the pulse rate recorded.

T-tube Cholangiogram

This is performed 7–10 days after operative removal of gall stones to check whether there are any residual stones. No sedation is necessary. Contrast medium is injected into the T-tube which has been left in the common bile duct to provide drainage and an x-ray is taken.

LIVER

The liver may be examined by:
1. Straight radiograph.
2. Angiogram (see p. 216).
3. Isotope scanning ('liver scan'). This can be used to show tumour masses in the liver.
4. ERCP (Endoscopic Retrograde Cholangio-Pancreatography). This enables the biliary tract to be visualised (see p. 27).

TEETH

X-ray examinations are frequently of value in dental conditions, and may show the following: apical abscess (an abscess at the root of a tooth); bone infection round teeth; dental cysts; unerupted teeth.

Bones, Joints and Tendons

The following methods of examination are used:
1. *Straight radiograph.*
2. *Arthrogram.* This is the injection of radio-opaque

material or air into a joint to outline the joint cavity on
x-ray.

3. *Bone scans* (p. 207). This is used mainly for secondary
tumours.

4. *Cineradiography.* A cine-film of the x-ray appearance of
the joint in movement provides accurate information concerning its function. Tendon function may similarly be
studied (see Tenogram, p. 215).

The conditions which may be demonstrated include:

Abscesses and cysts are visible, e.g. Brodie's abscess in the
upper end of the tibia.

Arthritis. Acute and chronic. In acute arthritis the bones
will be decalcified. In chronic arthritis the erosion of bone
and new formation of bone is seen. Ankylosis of the joint
may be demonstrated.

Dislocations and subluxations. The abnormal position of
the bone is seen. After the dislocation has been reduced, an
x-ray will confirm the fact that the position is now correct.

Fractures. An x-ray will demonstrate a fracture, and also its
type, e.g. comminuted, greenstick, impacted, spiral, etc. In
some situations skill is required to place the part in such a
position that the fracture will be visible, e.g. head of radius,
scaphoid, etc. After a fracture has been reduced, a further
x-ray will show whether or not the position is satisfactory.
Subsequently, an x-ray will show whether or not the fracture is united.

In a compound fracture with delayed healing due to
infection, an x-ray may show the presence of a sequestrum.

It is most important that all cases of injury where there is
any possibility of a fracture should have an x-ray
examination.

An x-ray of a fracture may reveal the fact that the bone is
broken at the side of a secondary growth, the presence of
which was not previously recognised. This is known as a
pathological fracture.

Growths of bones are visible on x-ray examination. They may be simple or malignant. A simple growth may be a chondroma, osteoma, etc. Malignant growths may be primary, e.g. osteosarcoma, or secondary, e.g. a secondary growth in the femur from carcinoma of the breast.

Osteomyelitis. In acute osteomyelitis some days must elapse after the onset of the disease before changes are visible on x-ray examination. In chronic osteomyelitis, a sequestrum is often visible or a Brodie's abscess may be seen.

Periostitis is visible on x-ray examination after the condition is well established.

Rickets. The changes of rickets are well shown on x-ray examination. Evidence is often obtained from the lower end of the radius.

Scurvy. In this condition haemorrhage occurs under the periosteum of bones in the neighbourhood of joints. This is visible in x-ray examination. The epiphyseal line is irregular.

Skull. Most fractures of the skull are visible on x-ray examination. Bony conditions giving rise to Jacksonian fits may be demonstrable.

An enlarged pituitary fossa is suggestive of a pituitary tumour, or chronic raised intracranial pressure.

Tenogram. Injections of radio-opaque material into a tendon sheath enables the tendon and its sheath to be clearly visualised on x-ray, and its function studied by cine-radiography (see p. 214).

Tuberculosis of bones and joints. These conditions may be diagnosed by the x-ray picture. The course of the disease is verified by x-ray examinations at various stages of the illness. The formation of abscesses, necrotic bone, and the ultimate bony ankylosis are all demonstrable.

Various bone diseases show diagnostic changes on x-ray examination. Among these may be mentioned achondroplasia, fibrocystic disease, fragilitas ossium, Paget's disease, Perthe's disease and osteomalacia.

Measurements of female pelvis. See p. 221.

Cardiovascular System

Heart. The heart is clearly visible on x-ray examination and the heart size can be assessed. In certain types of heart disease the heart assumes definite shapes, e.g. boot-shape in hypertension. Calcification is sometimes seen in valvular disease and pericarditis. A pericardial effusion can be demonstrated.

Aneurysms of large vessels are sometimes visible on straight x-ray but are better shown on angiogram. Ultrasound is also useful for demonstrating abdominal aneurysms.

Angiography. Injection of radio-opaque dye into a vessel and rapid filming provides an angiogram. This outlines the vessel showing any obstruction, aneurysm or abnormal course. An angiogram of the aorta is called an aortogram, of arteries an arteriogram and of veins a venogram or phlebogram. A number of specialised investigations may be undertaken, e.g. splenic venogram, hepatic arteriogram or renal arteriogram, which outline the vasculature in the respective organs. Abnormal vessels may be demonstrated in tumours of the viscera and obstruction of arteries seen, e.g. in the legs in cases of intermittent claudication. (See also angiogram of cerebral vessels, p. 222.)

Angiocardiography. See p. 109.

Lymphangiography. Certain lymph nodes and vessels can be demonstrated by injection of ultra-fluid Lipiodol through a tiny cannula into a lymph vessel in the dorsum of the foot to produce a lymphangiogram. This is of value in showing lymph node involvement in pelvic carcinoma and Hodgkin's disease.

To locate the fine lymphatics in the feet a blue dye is injected between the toes. For a few hours after the procedure the patient may appear blue and the urine become green. The examination takes at least three hours and is tedious for both patient and radiologist. The injected oil eventually enters the neck veins and reaches the lungs where it temporarily impairs function. It is contra-indicated in patients with severe lung disease.

Respiratory System

X-ray examinations include:

1. *Straight radiographs* of chest (postero-anterior and lateral) and of sinuses.

2. *Tomography*. This is a technique for obtaining a radiographic 'section' (usually coronal) of the chest at a given depth. It is of value in investigating a small tumour or cavity.

3. *Screening*. The lungs and their movements are observed by a fluoroscopic screen placed in front of the patient via an image intensifier and television link.

4. *Bronchography*. The bronchial tree may be clearly outlined by the introduction of contrast medium. It is used for the diagnosis of bronchiectasis and other bronchial abnormalities, e.g. tumours. About 10ml of medium is injected, the patient meanwhile lying on the side which it is desired to show, so that the medium will run by gravity into the lung concerned. It runs into the lower bronchioles, rendering them opaque to x-rays. This shows up dilatation from bronchiectasis or constriction from a tumour.

A laryngeal catheter is passed through the nose to the larynx and radio-opaque medium injected through this.

5. *Lung scans*, using radio-isotopes.

6. *Miniature mass radiography*. By using miniature films, population surveys may be carried out at a relatively small cost. Suspect cases are then examined using full-size films.

The following are examples of conditions which may be demonstrated:

Abscess of the lung. A cavity, perhaps with a fluid level, is seen.

Bronchiectasis. Certain changes are visible on a straight x-ray, but the bronchial dilatations are better demonstrated by a bronchogram.

Pleural effusion and empyema. An opacity is seen, perhaps with a fluid level, which can be seen to move with respiration and posture on screen examination.

Fibroid lung. The collapsed lung is visible, and possibly some displacement of the heart which is pulled over by the contraction of the lung.

Growths. These are visible and may be primary or secondary. Primary growths may be carcinoma of the lung, or mediastinal tumours. Secondary growths may be deposits of sarcoma or carcinoma from primary growths in other parts of the body.

Enlarged mediastinal glands in Hodgkin's disease may be seen.

Hydatid cysts have a typical circular appearance with clear-cut edges, and possibly a fluid level.

Pneumonia. The consolidation of pneumonia gives an opacity on the radiograph.

Pneumothorax. Air in the pleural cavity is seen as a space free from lung markings around the collapsed lung.

Silicosis. This gives the lung shadow a characteristic mottled appearance.

Tuberculosis. X-ray examination is of great value in pulmonary tuberculosis. In early cases it is an essential aid to diagnosis. In later stages it is of value in assessing the response to treatment. Areas of infiltration, calcification, cavities, air, fluid, or pus in the pleural cavity are all visible. The height of the diaphragm is raised after crushing of the phrenic nerve. Miliary tuberculosis gives an appearance likened to a snowstorm. Tuberculous mediastinal glands may also be seen.

Nasal sinuses. Disease of these structures renders them opaque.

Urogenital System

A straight x-ray may show the presence of a calculus in the kidneys, ureters, or bladder.

Other procedures are:

INTRAVENOUS PYELOGRAM (IVP, also called Intravenous Urography, IVU)

When a suitable contrast medium is injected intravenously it is excreted by functioning kidneys, rendering the urinary tract opaque to x-rays.

The night before the examination the patient should be given liquid extract of cascara, and the following morning a high enema about an hour or so before the examination. It is important for this procedure to eliminate gas in the intestines as this interferes with the definition of the radiograph. In addition fluids are not given for some hours prior to the examination (to render the urine more concentrated) and the bladder is emptied just before the commencement. A contrast medium, e.g. 15–40ml of sodium diatrizoate (45 per cent w/v) is injected intravenously and films are taken after 5 minutes, 10 minutes, and 20 minutes.

When the urinary tract is obstructed delayed films may be required, possibly on the following day, as the obstructed kidney only excretes slowly. The test can be used in acute or chronic renal failure but the patient should not be dehydrated beforehand and high doses of contrast medium may be required.

The IVP is a valuable test of kidney function. It also demonstrates hydronephrosis, hypernephroma, calculi, etc.

RETROGRADE PYELOGRAM

The preparation of the patient is similar to that for an intravenous pyelogram but without restriction of fluids.

A cystoscope is passed, and a ureteric catheter inserted into each ureter. A solution of Hypaque is then injected up each ureteric catheter. The quantity that the renal pelvis will hold varies according to the condition present, and the injection is stopped when the patient complains of a pain in the loin. Sodium iodide is opaque to x-rays and when a film is taken the ureter, renal pelvis, and calyces will be shown. This procedure is useful for demonstrating calculi, hydronephrosis, hypernephroma, etc.

CYSTOGRAM

This usually forms part of the IVP, described above, as the contrast medium collects in the bladder, providing an outline of the organ on a radiograph. More controlled bladder filling is obtained using a catheter, retrograde cystography. This can be of particular value to see whether there is fluid reflux up the ureters during micturition (micturating cystogram) which may be an important factor in producing recurrent pyelonephritis.

UTERUS, TUBES AND OVARIES

Because of the possible damaging effects of radiation to the developing fetus, abdominal radiography on female patients of child-bearing age is now avoided except in the first 10 days of the menstrual cycle (the 'ten-day rule').

A straight x-ray may show a dermoid cyst, containing teeth or bony structures. A calcified fibroid tumour may also be seen.

Pregnancy

The use of x-rays during pregnancy has been greatly reduced as a result of the recognition that irradiation may be harmful to the growing fetus, possibly promoting leukaemia on occasions. They are no longer used to demonstrate fetal bones in doubtful cases of pregnancy. Measurement of the diameters of the pelvis (pelvimetry) by means of x-rays has been reduced to the minimum.

However, in carefully selected cases x-rays are still of considerable value. They are used to demonstrate abnormalities of the fetus such as anencephaly and hydrocephalus; fetal death by the overlapping of the cranial bones; doubtful positions, e.g. ? breech presentation; the presence of twins or triplets; also fetal maturity determination and the demonstration of abnormalities by means of a placentogram.

Ultrasound (p. 208), is now being used to replace x-rays in estimating fetal maturity, measuring the biparietal diameter and for detecting multiple births, fetal abnormalities and placental site. Pelvic organs can be seen better when the bladder is full. So the patient is given three glasses of water to drink before examination.

Salpingogram

In the female, sterility may be due to the fact that the Fallopian tubes are not patent. To test the patency, a special syringe is inserted into the cervical os, and contrast medium injected. An x-ray photograph is then taken by which it can be seen whether the passage of the medium is obstructed in the tube or is dripping through the fimbriated end into the abdominal cavity.

Breast and Soft Tissues

MAMMOGRAPHY

Soft tissue x-rays are passed through the breast only, with the patient in the erect and supine positions. By using low kilovoltage x-rays, a clearer picture of soft tissue changes is obtained. Microcalcification can be detected in a small cancer before it can be detected clinically by palpation.

XERORADIOGRAPHY (Xerography)

This is a medical application of the photocopying process. It enables the clarity of soft tissue x-rays to be enhanced, with the production of a blue photocopy.

THERMOGRAPHY

Heat given out from the body in the form of infra-red emission can be recorded to detect 'hot spots'. These indicate possible sites of cancer. Thermography is not sufficiently specific to be a diagnostic technique, but may be used for screening, prior to mammography.

Nervous System

ANGIOGRAM

Abnormal conditions of the cerebral vessels, e.g. aneurysms, can be demonstrated by injecting a contrast medium, e.g. sodium diatrizoate, rapidly into the carotid artery in the neck. This procedure is not free from risk but may be an essential preoperative investigation.

ENCEPHALOGRAM

A lumbar puncture is performed with the patient in a sitting posture, and some cerebrospinal fluid is allowed to escape. About 50 to 90ml of air are then injected through the lumbar puncture needle. This ascends to the cavities in the brain, and their outline will be seen on a radiograph. The photograph is taken with the patient lying down, and the head in special positions.

A method is also available in which only a small quantity of air, about 5 to 10ml, is injected and photographs taken after tilting the head in various positions.

This procedure is useful in cases of cerebral tumour.

MYELOGRAM

The spinal cord can be examined by the injection of Myodil into the space between the meninges and the cord (sub-arachnoid space). A lumbar puncture is performed (see p. 127). With the patient sitting, 5–8ml of Myodil is injected into the subarachnoid space. The patient is then placed on a tilting table and screened. By tilting the patient the Myodil can be made to move up or down. If an obstruction or filling defect is demonstrated (e.g. due to a tumour), films are taken.

VENTRICULOGRAM

A small hole is bored through the skull in the parietal region, and a special cannula inserted through the cortex into the lateral ventricle. Some cerebrospinal fluid is allowed to escape, and then about 20–30ml of air are injected. On x-ray examination the outline of the ventricle will be seen. This procedure is useful in cases of cerebral tumour.

BRAIN SCANS

Intravenous injection of radio-isotopes is now frequently used to demonstrate space-occupying lesions in the brain, such as tumours or haematomata, and reducing the need for other investigations. Ultrasound scans may also be used, e.g. to demonstrate a shift of the midline of the brain.

Foreign Bodies

These can be demonstrated if opaque to x-rays. Methods of examination include:

1. *Straight radiographs.*

2. *Stereoradiography.* The stereoscope is an instrument whereby two x-ray photographs taken from slightly different positions enable a three-dimensional x-ray picture to be obtained. This procedure may help in the localisation of a foreign body.

3. *Sinogram.* In some cases contrast medium may be injected down a chronic sinus and an x-ray examination carried out to ascertain its extent.

Alimentary tract. Articles may be swallowed by children or adults. If by adults it may be by accident or by intention (attempted suicide and in mental disorders). Such articles may be coins, portions of dentures, pieces of bones, buttons, pins, safety-pins, cutlery, buckles, etc, etc.

The size of the article may indicate whether removal is advisable or not. If there is a probability of the object passing through the alimentary tract without injury, later photographs can be taken indicating its progress.

Foreign bodies may also be introduced into the rectum occasionally.

Aural and nasal cavities. Foreign bodies may be introduced here by children. An x-ray may be advisable in some cases of a chronic discharge.

Respiratory system. Small foreign bodies which are inhaled may pass into the larynx and thence to the bronchi. Such articles may be teeth, portions of dentures, small beads, fragments of toys, etc. X-ray examination may localise the object prior to bronchoscopy.

Urogenital system. Foreign bodies may be introduced into the bladders of children and occasionally of adult females.

Objects may be lodged in the uterus or surrounding structures in cases of criminal abortion.

Penetrating wounds. Foreign bodies may be found in any structure of the body as a result of their entrance through the skin surface, e.g. needles, bullets, etc. Any such object may be found a considerable distance from where it has gained entrance.

Once a foreign body is seen, it is necessary to have accurate localisation to facilitate its removal. For this purpose photographs from different angles are taken, and its position estimated from known bony structures. See also Stereoradiography (p. 224).

Skin sinuses and fistulae. In some cases of a chronic sinus opening on to the skin surface, it may be necessary for an x-ray to be taken to see if there is a foreign body present preventing healing. See Sinogram (p. 224).

SECTION NINE
Miscellaneous Tests

Miscellaneous Tests

Infections

Blood tests used in the diagnosis of infections are described under Bacteriological Tests on Blood, p. 73.

under Bacteriological Tests on Blood, p. 73.

WOUNDS, ABSCESSES, DISCHARGES AND INFECTED FLUIDS

Before starting treatment of a septic condition it is important to send a specimen of the infected material to the laboratory so that the causative organism may be identified and tested for sensitivity to antibacterial drugs. Pus should be collected into a sterile container, if present in sufficient quantity. If not, a sterile swab should be taken. Exceptionally, e.g. with discharges from actinomycotic sinuses, it may be necessary to send the dressings to the laboratory in an appropriate sterile receptacle. For vaginal and urethral discharges see p. 168, and for urinary infection, p. 152. For septicaemia, blood cultures are required (p. 73). In meningitis the cerebrospinal fluid is examined (p. 127).

TYPE OF SWAB TO USE

The swabs commonly used in most hospitals are (a) serum coated, (b) charcoal and (c) alginate. **Serum coated swabs** are the ones generally used, e.g. for nasal, throat, wound, pus swabs etc. **Charcoal swabs** are used for suspected gonococcal infection but must not be used for eye infections of the new born (ophthalmia neonatorum) for which a platinum loop is usually used (see Eye Swabs, p. 231). **Alginate swabs** are used almost entirely for laryngeal swabs when TB is suspected. Many micro-organisms die very quickly (especially gonococci and the anaerobic organisms, e.g. bacteroides, etc), if allowed to dry or are exposed to air for more than a very short time. So transport medium should be used if any delay is anticipated.

NB It is better to send pus in a sterile container rather than swabs whenever possible. Similarly, a specimen of stool in a universal container is better than a stool swab.

TRANSPORT MEDIA

This should be used if there is a possibility of any delay between taking the specimen from the patient and sending it to the laboratory, viz (a) Virus transport medium; (b) Stuart's medium; (c) Trichomonas medium; (d) Other transport media. **Virus transport medium** is a balanced salt solution containing antibiotics used for throat swabs, mouth washings, etc, when virus infection is suspected. **Stuart's medium** is excellent for most bacteriological infections. It is a clear thick fluid containing reducing substances to prevent anaerobic bacteria from dying. **Trichomonas medium** is a dark brown fluid used for isolating trichomonas and candida (monilia) from vaginal swabs, etc. **Other transport media** include cytomegalovirus (CMV) medium which is similar to virus transport medium but contains a special sugar (sorbitol) and should be used when transporting urine or throat swabs for suspected CMV infections, mainly in infants.

SPECIMENS FROM PATIENTS WITH TRANSMISSIBLE
INFECTIONS

When collecting or handling specimens from patients who are Australia antigen positive or who have other transmissible infections, e.g. typhoid or bacillary dysentery, take the following precautions. Protective clothing should be worn viz disposable gown and gloves. For a case of open tuberculosis, a mask should be worn. Do not squirt fluid through a fine needle as this produces an aerosol. Avoid spillage. Treat any spilt fluid immediately with strong hypochlorite or 2% activated glutaraldehyde. Place specimen containers in individual plastic bags marked with coloured 'High Risk' stickers. Put a similar sticker on the request form. Use sticky tape to seal the bags, not staples, ensuring that neither container nor bag can leak. Dispose of needles and syringes into safe receptacles. Report any accident or mishap immediately.

For highly infectious diseases, e.g. haemorrhagic virus diseases such as Lassa fever, some of the above recommendations may need to be modified in the light of the isolation unit's own code of practice.

ASSAY OF ANTIBACTERIAL DRUGS

Occasionally it is of value to collect samples of blood or other fluids to estimate the level of antibacterial substances present. 5ml of blood, or other fluid, should be collected into a sterile container. This procedure is necessary when testing new drugs, when the presence of kidney damage could lead to toxic blood levels and when monitoring progress during long periods of treatment for certain infections, e.g. endocarditis.

EYE SWABS

These are taken prior to operations on the eye and also in cases of infections of the eye. It is best for the swab to be taken by the laboratory staff at the bedside. A platinum loop is used which is sterilised by flaming. The upper lid is held firmly to prevent blinking and the lower lid everted. The swab is then taken from the conjunctiva over the lower anterior surface of the sclera.

It is most important that the swab does not touch the eyelids. The swab is then spread directly on to a 'chocolate' blood agar plate, which is then incubated for 48 hours or more. If organisms such as the Staphylococcus aureus or β-haemolytic streptococcus are present, any ophthalmic operation must be postponed until the infection is cleared.

FUNGAL INFECTIONS OF SKIN, INCLUDING RINGWORM

Skin scrapings and damaged hairs from the affected area should be sent to the laboratory in a dry sterile container where the fungus can be identified by microscopy and culture. Wood's glass is a coloured filter placed in front of an ultra-violet lamp. This is used sometimes in the diagnosis of ringworm or the confirmation of its cure. If the light is shone on to a suspected area, hairs affected by ringworm show up in a fluorescent manner. It is not an infallible test.

VIRUS AND RICKETTSIAL INFECTIONS

Viruses and Rickettsiae can be isolated by culture, but more often their presence is inferred by the demonstration of increasing amounts of antibody in the patient's blood. In certain virus and rickettsial infections microscopy is of value in demonstrating inclusion bodies inside the patient's cells.

Culture

Viruses can be grown only in living tissue, usually in the form of a tissue culture or in the developing membranes of a chick embryo. They will not grow like bacteria in simple culture broths. Poliomyelitis for example can be isolated from faeces using a tissue culture of monkey kidney epithelium: influenza virus can be isolated in a chick embryo from throat washings of a patient. This is of great value in identifying the type of virus in an epidemic but is too slow for routine diagnosis.

Rickettsiae which cause typhus fever can also be grown in a developing chick embryo, but are usually first isolated by inoculating the blood of a fresh case into the peritoneal cavity of a guinea-pig.

Antibody demonstration

Two samples are required, each about 5ml of clotted blood, the first early in the disease, the second late or during convalescence. The second sample shows at least a four-fold increase in titre of antibody against a particular virus or rickettsia if this has caused the disease. This is the most widely used diagnostic method in virology.

Weil-Felix reaction

The blood from a patient with typhus contains antibody which agglutinates a strain of proteus.

Microscopy

Viruses cannot be seen as separate particles by the ordinary microscope, only by the electron microscope. Rickettsiae are slightly larger and are just visible under the ordinary light microscope, especially if present in large numbers. In certain virus and rickettsial diseases, bodies visible under the ordinary microscope appear inside the cells, known as inclusion bodies. They may be seen in smears from the eyelids in acute trachoma or in swimming-pool conjunctivitis, also in brain sections from dogs with rabies.

Electron microscopy

In some centres it is becoming a practical proposition to make a diagnosis of the type of virus causing an infection by recognition of its shape under the electron microscope. This can be of immense value, e.g. in the early diagnosis of smallpox by examination of pustular fluid.

Diagnostic Skin Tests

In the following intradermal skin tests a positive result implies sensitivity to a particular protein, either from an infecting organism or else some other foreign protein. Certain tests in which a positive result has a different implication (viz Schick, Dick and Scarlet fever blanching test) are described under the heading 'Other Types of Diagnostic Skin Test' (p. 238).

NB Diagnostic skin tests are now rarely used apart from the tuberculin and Kveim test. Cat-scratch antigen is often not available although the test itself is useful.

CASONI TEST

This is a test for hydatid disease. It is no longer performed in the United Kingdom. (See p. 77.)

Sterile hydatid fluid is obtainable in a small ampoule from the Public Health Laboratory and 0.2ml of this is injected intradermally. A control is provided by injecting the same quantity of sheep's serum at another site.

A positive reaction occurs when a white weal up to 5cm in diameter, with pseudopodia, surrounded by erythema, appears at the site of the injection of hydatid fluid. The reaction appears within 20 minutes, and fades in an hour or two. Dermal induration is present after 24 hours.

The test is positive in some 90 per cent of cases of hydatid disease. It does, however, remain positive for many years after a hydatid cyst has been removed.

CAT-SCRATCH FEVER

Antigen, prepared from an affected lymph node of a known case of this disease, is obtainable (but not often available) from the Public Health Laboratory and 0.2ml is injected intradermally. A positive result is a firm red area at least 1cm in diameter appearing in 48 hours and persisting sometimes for several weeks. It implies present or previous cat-scratch fever.

COCCIDIOIDIN

Coccidioidin is the antigen prepared from the fungus Coccidioides immitis which causes coccidioidomycosis and 0.2ml of the antigen preparation is injected intradermally. A positive result is a firm red area at least 1cm in diameter within 48–72 hours. It implies present or previous infection.

FREI TEST (see p. 169)

HISTOPLASMIN

Histoplasmin is the antigen prepared from the fungus Histoplasma capsulatum which causes histoplasmosis. The skin test is performed as for coccidioidin (p. 234). A positive result implies present or previous infection.

KVEIM TEST

This is a test for sarcoidosis. The Kveim antigen, available from the Public Health Laboratory, is injected intradermally. Several weeks later a small swelling appears at the site. A biopsy specimen of the swelling is taken into formalin for histology. In a positive result there are microscopic changes typical of sarcoidosis. This implies that the patient has sarcoidosis.

SERUM SENSITISATION

Some persons develop an undue sensitivity to serum or antitoxin once an injection has been given. In such cases a second injection of serum may produce the reaction known as anaphylaxis which may be serious or even fatal. To avoid this, a test for serum sensitisation is performed when it is necessary to give serum to persons who may have had it previously. A small quantity of serum, about 0.25–0.5ml, is injected intradermally and the result observed. If the person is sensitive a red urticarial patch occurs at the site of injection within an hour or so. In such cases serum must be administered in small doses spread over several hours.

SKIN REACTIONS FOR HYPERSENSITIVITY

Certain persons are unduly sensitive to certain proteins, and various conditions may be set up by exposure to them. Among such conditions are asthma, skin rashes, and hay fever. The proteins which may cause these reactions are many, e.g. grass pollen, hairs of animals, certain foods, etc. Preparations of the proteins are sold by commercial firms.

In order to test a patient several of a similar type are formed into a group. A series of small scratches are made on the forearm, and a small quantity of each group rubbed into a different scratch mark, by means of a glass rod. Alternatively the preparations may be injected intradermally. A positive reaction is shown by the development of a reddish area with a weal in about 15 to 20 minutes.

If one particular group gives a positive reaction, further tests may be carried out employing the individual members of the group.

These tests are not very accurate, and often multiple positive reactions are given. If, however, any particular type gives a reaction, the patient should avoid exposure to the article in question, or be desensitised—if possible.

TRICHINA ANTIGEN TEST

This is a test for trichinosis, a condition in which the muscles are invaded by the larvae of the parasite Trichinella spiralis. The test is carried out as for coccidioidin (p. 234). A positive result implies that the patient has trichinosis.

Tuberculin Skin Reactions

A positive tuberculin skin reaction indicates that the subject has at some time been infected by the tubercle bacillus. Although it is really a test for sensitivity to tuberculin, it is taken to indicate that the person has some degree of immunity against tuberculosis. It does not indicate whether or not active infection is present. A negative reaction indicates an absence of immunity to tuberculosis. This is usually because the person has not been exposed to tuberculous infection and is therefore susceptible; it may very occasionally be found in a person with active infection who is without any immunity.

Immunity may be conferred by inoculation with BCG (Bacillus Calmette-Guérin), a harmless form of the tubercle bacillus. If successful, the tuberculin reaction which was previously negative becomes positive within 6 weeks of immunisation.

MANTOUX TEST

This is the most reliable tuberculin skin reaction and the one in common use. A small quantity of tuberculin is injected intradermally, using old tuberculin or tuberculin purified protein derivative (PPD) in a dilution of 1 in 1 000. An intradermal injection of 0.1ml is given on the flexor surface of the forearm. Normal saline may be used as a control at another site. If the test is positive a red area appears at the site of injection, reaching its maximum at 48 hours. If no reaction occurs, the test is repeated using tuberculin diluted 1 in 100. In patients who may have active tuberculous infection, the first test should be done using tuberculin at a dilution of 1 in 10 000 to avoid the possibility of a serious general reaction.

A variant of the Mantoux test is the multiple puncture technique (Heaf test). Instead of using a syringe a special instrument with a number of points is used to introduce the tuberculin intradermally. An alternative is the tine test.

PATCH TEST

This is more convenient for babies, but is not so reliable and may give false negative reactions.

A small patch containing tuberculin is stuck on the skin, usually on the back, for 48 hours. A control area is included in the patch. After 48 hours the result is read. A positive result is similar to that for the Mantoux test.

VON PIRQUET'S TEST

The skin of the forearm is cleansed. Two drops of the tuberculin testing solution are placed on the skin about

10cm apart, and between them a drop of normal saline is placed as a control. The skin is scarified through the drops. The drops are wiped off after 10 minutes. If the test is positive a papule at least 1cm in diameter forms, reaching its maximum in 48 hours.

Other Types of Diagnostic Skin Test

SCHICK TEST

This test is used to ascertain whether a person is susceptible to diphtheria. 0.2ml of the diluted diphtheria toxin, specially prepared for the Schick Test, is injected intradermally into the flexor surface of the forearm. A control injection of heated toxin into the other arm is used as a comparison.

If there is, in 24 to 48 hours, a red area about 2.5cm wide, the reaction is positive, and the person is susceptible to diphtheria. If there is no red area, or if there is a slight reaction equal in both arms, the test is negative, and the person is not susceptible to diphtheria.

The test is also used in doubtful cases of diphtheria, the majority of such cases giving a positive test. Later in the disease the test becomes negative.

The test is also of value in examination of persons who are contacts in a diphtheria epidemic—they may be thus divided into those who may develop the disease, and those who probably will not.

Persons found to be susceptible to diphtheria may be protected against it by means of immunising injections. This procedure has been carried out to a considerable extent in children in an attempt to eradicate the disease, with notable success.

DICK TEST

This is performed in a similar manner to the Schick test. A small quantity of scarlet fever toxin is injected intradermally, and a red area indicates a positive reaction, and the fact that the person is susceptible to scarlet fever. It is not so reliable as the Schick test.

SCARLET FEVER BLANCHING TEST

Into an area of skin affected by the rash 0.2ml of a 1 in 10 dilution of scarlet fever antitoxin is injected intradermally. If a zone of blanching appears within 24 hours and persists, the rash is scarlatinal. This is sometimes called the Schultz-Charlton reaction and the test is only occasionally used.

Prevention of Infection

AIR CONTAMINATION

The degree of air contamination by organisms can be measured by a slit sampler (Bordillon). This sucks in air at a controlled rate over a rotating blood agar plate. The organisms stick to the surface and after incubation the bacterial colonies are counted. It is becoming a standard method of checking the degree of air contamination in the ward and operating theatre.

Culture plates, exposed to the air, are also used to determine the number of bacteria-carrying particles settling on the surface over a known time interval. By counting the number of colonies on the plates after incubation, the number of bacteria-carrying particles can be estimated.

STERILITY OF DRESSINGS

Five tests are in common use to check whether the sterilisation of dressing drums is adequate.
1. Spore strips containing spores of B. stearothermophilus can be inserted in the dressing drum prior to sterilisation. At the completion of sterilisation, efforts to grow organisms from the spore strip should be unsuccessful.
2. A small tube (Browne's tube) containing a red liquid

may be placed in a drum of dressings prior to sterilisation. After sufficient time at the required temperature the liquid turns green. Amber ('caution') implies inadequate sterilisation. Old tubes may change colour after inadequate heat exposure or even without any exposure to heat. So it is important to use only fresh tubes.

3. Bowie Dick test for high vacuum sterilisers is now in common use. A batch of a dozen surgical towels is taken and to one of the central towels two strips of special tape (made by the Minnesota Mining Co) are stuck in the form of a St Andrew's cross. After sterilisation the brown bands which develop on the tape must be present at the site of intersection.

4. Paper which changes colour, e.g. Klintex autoclave test paper is not so reliable but does provide evidence that the drum has been exposed to heat.

5. Thermocouple. The insertion of a thermocouple into the material being sterilised is a very reliable method of measuring the temperature. It is not convenient for the daily routine but should be used on commissioning a new autoclave, after repairs and also at 6-monthly intervals.

TEST FOR BLANKET CONTAMINATION

For this test sterile salt agar in a Petri dish is provided by the laboratory. Immediately before sampling, the cover of the Petri dish is removed. The base of the Petri dish containing the salt agar is inverted over the blanket. Six sweeps are made across the surface of the blanket. The edge of the Petri dish roughs up the blanket and any organisms tend to be brushed up on to the surface of the agar. The cover is replaced. The Petri dish is labelled and returned to the laboratory. The test is of value in making random checks on ward blankets in use and also as a check on the sterility of blankets which have been sterilised.

MILK

Milk has to be of a certain standard, and tests are carried out for the following purposes:

1. To estimate the fat content and so detect any adulteration with water.

2. To estimate the bacterial content and the possible presence of any bacteria which should not be present.

Only two special types of milk, pasteurised and sterilised, are marketed in England and Wales. Tuberculin-tested milk is no longer specially designated since the whole of England, Scotland and Wales is now an attested area in which all cattle are tested to see that they are free from tuberculosis.

Formerly tuberculin-tested milk had to fail to decolourise methylene blue within $4\frac{1}{2}$ hours in summer and $5\frac{1}{2}$ hours in winter. The rate of decolourisation of methylene blue depends on the number of bacteria present.

Pasteurised milk

This is milk which has been heated to a temperature of 63°C for half an hour (or using the High Temperature Short Time method, 72°C for 20 seconds) and immediately cooled to less than 10°C. This destroys most of the bacteria. Pasteurised milk must give a 'negative' phosphatase test (2.3 Lovibond units or less). Phosphatase is an enzyme which occurs normally in milk and which is practically destroyed by adequate pasteurisation.

In addition a sample of pasteurised milk which is taken on the day of delivery and kept below 18°C should, until 0900–10.00 of the day following delivery, fail to decolourise methylene blue in 30 minutes.

Sterilised milk

The milk is filtered, homogenised and heated to a temperature of at least 100°C for sufficient time to comply with the turbidity test. The bottles are sealed with airtight seals.

After sterilisation the milk should show no turbidity on testing.

Infection in milk
Certain diseases may be transmitted by milk, e.g. tuberculosis, scarlet fever, epidemic diarrhoea, abortus fever, undulant fever, typhoid fever, diphtheria. In some cases the milk is infected by 'carriers' who handle it.

Examination of Tissues (Histology)

Biopsy

By this is meant that some tissue is taken from a patient and examined microscopically. This frequently enables a correct diagnosis to be made. It is of particular value in determining whether a tumour is malignant or not, and the treatment to be adopted often depends on the result of the histological examination.

A small portion of the tissue in question is placed in a small bottle containing 10% formalin in saline or other fixative, which is accurately labelled and sent to the laboratory. There it is hardened and mounted in a wax block from which thin sections are cut, stained and examined microscopically. A report is normally available in a few days.

FROZEN SECTION

A more rapid method is available using a freezing process which provides a result within 5 to 10 minutes. This method can be used during the course of an operation, e.g. a portion of a tumour from the breast can be examined at the commencement of an operation, and on receipt of the report some minutes later the extent of the operation can be determined. The pathologist is notified in advance to ensure that he is available. The tissue for examination is placed in a dry container and sent to the histology laboratory as quickly as possible. Then the pathologist selects an appropriate small block of tissue. The technician freezes the tissue on to a holder (chuck) by means of compressed carbon dioxide from a cylinder. He then cuts sections using a microtome which is either cooled by carbon dioxide (freezing microtome) or placed inside a refrigerated cabinet (cryostat). The sections are put on slides, stained rapidly and then examined by the pathologist who telephones the result to the operating theatre. Frozen sections are also used to demonstrate fats (lipids) and enzymes which would be destroyed by the ordinary processing methods.

Special Types of Biopsy

ASPIRATION BIOPSY

Tissue may be punctured with an aspiration biopsy needle and the small cylinder of material aspirated sent to the laboratory for examination. This may be done in diseases of the liver (p. 23), kidney (p. 159), spleen, bone marrow (p. 51) and pleura. It often provides valuable information and may be diagnostic.

BIOPSY OF ENDOMETRIUM

A small amount of endometrium is removed with a special instrument and sent to the laboratory for report. This can be done in the outpatient department. It is useful in the diagnosis of growths of the uterus, disorders of menstruation, etc (see Uterine Curettings, p. 167).

BIOPSY OF TESTIS (see p. 166)

BIOPSY OF SKIN AND LYMPH NODES

Skin lesions and enlarged lymph nodes (preferably not groin glands) can be removed for histological diagnosis.

BIOPSY OF STOMACH

A portion of tissue, e.g. from an ulcer suspected of malignancy is taken from the stomach through a gastroscope (see p. 12).

BIOPSY OF SMALL INTESTINE (see p. 31)

BLADDER BIOPSY

A portion of bladder wall bearing a papilloma or other lesion is removed through a cystoscope (see p. 159).

BONE BIOPSY

This is used in the diagnosis of bone tumours and other bone diseases, e.g. cysts, Paget's disease and osteomalacia. The bone specimen is usually obtained by open operation and collected into formal saline. Sometimes a small cylinder can be obtained using a trephine through an aspiration biopsy needle (see bone marrow puncture, p. 51). Where osteomalacia is suspected the specimen should be collected into *neutral* formal saline (ordinary formalin, if acid, tends to remove calcium from the bone).

BRONCHIAL BIOPSY

Portions of tumour and other lesions of the bronchus can be removed by bronchoscopy (p. 120).

Examination of Cells (Cytology)

Exfoliative Cytology

This is the study of shed cells. Cancer cells usually have a different microscopic appearance from normal cells. This enables certain types of cancer, e.g. of the cervix uteri, to be diagnosed at an early stage. To make the proper diagnosis on any smear, it is extremely important that all the technical details be performed with care. It is easier to prepare smears if the proper equipment is at hand, usually available from the cytology department. Particular attention should be paid to spreading the smear evenly, not too thickly (nor too thinly), and fixing while still wet. Fixatives are of several kinds. Some are sprayed on, some are poured on and some the slides are immersed in, e.g. alcohol fixative. With the latter there must be at least sufficient fixative to cover all the smear, and the lid must be replaced on the container to prevent evaporation.

CERVICAL AND VAGINAL CYTOLOGY (see Papanicolaou smear, p. 167)

SPUTUM

The specimen must be fresh and coughed from 'deep down'. It should be collected into a wide-mouthed container and sent to the laboratory within 2 hours. For the detection of cancer cells fresh unfixed sputum is very satisfactory. For the diagnosis of asthma the sputum should be collected into alcoholic fixative.

BRONCHIAL ASPIRATE

During bronchoscopy material can be sucked from the bronchus into a glass suction trap by washing the bronchi with 1–2ml of saline or on a cotton-wool plug in the aspirator itself. If secretion is scanty two slides should be prepared immediately and fixed while wet. Cytology may reveal cancer cells when the tumour is beyond the reach of the biopsy forceps.

GASTRIC CYTOLOGY

Gastric brush cytology has now virtually replaced gastric washout specimens (see Gastroscopy, p. 12).

PANCREATIC CYTOLOGY

Fluid from the pancreatic duct obtained by ERCP (p. 27) provides cytological material on which the diagnosis of a pancreatic tumour may be made.

PLEURAL AND PERITONEAL FLUIDS

The fluid should be sent to the laboratory immediately after being aspirated. Freshly aspirated fluid is examined for the types of cell present, e.g. leucocytes, red blood cells or cancer cells.

URINE

Freshly voided urine should be sent at once to the cytology laboratory. If this is not possible it should be immediately preserved by the addition of 50% alcohol. It is a sensitive method of detecting cancer cells of the urinary tract. It may also be used to detect the abnormal cells of inclusion body disease.

Other Applications of Cytology

BRAIN SMEARS

These can assist the surgeon to assess a brain tumour in the course of an operation.

SEX CHROMATIN

This is a structure present in the nuclei of normal female cells. It is related to the presence of two X chromosomes and enables the nuclear sex to be determined in herma-phrodites and other forms of intersex. One or more of the following are used:

1. Buccal squames
The inside of the cheek is scraped with a wooden spatula and smeared across a prepared (albuminised) glass slide. This is placed in fixative (alcohol ether).

2. *Blood films*

In females more than 1 per cent of the polymorphs contain 'drumstick' structures. Occasionally the results of this method do not agree with the others.

3. *Tissue sections*

Good histological sections of almost any tissue may be used, e.g. skin biopsy.

Chromosome Study

This gives more detailed information of the chromosome structure than sex chromatin examination (see above), but can only be done in special centres. A tissue culture from blood or bone marrow is often used.

Tissue Enzyme Study

The SAS tissue enzyme service has three aims:

1. Diagnosis of inherited metabolic diseases by assay of relevant enzymes in the appropriate cells, tissue or fluid.
2. Identification of carriers of the diseases by demonstration of partial enzyme deficiencies.
3. Prenatal diagnosis in high risk pregnancies for those diseases where adequate techniques are available.

Appropriate specimens include amniotic fluid (ideally from 15 weeks gestation), blood, skin and other tissues, depending on the enzymes to be studied. The SAS centre should be contacted and the case discussed before any tissues are collected. The SAS Tissue Enzyme Service is based at the Paediatric Research Unit, Prince Philip Research Laboratories, Guy's Hospital Medical School, London SE1 9RT Telephone 01-407 7600 Ext. 2342.

Other Miscellaneous Tests

MALINGERING

Symptoms are described inaccurately and in a different manner on repeated questionings.

Haemoptysis

The mouth and throat are examined for a self-inflicted injury. Also the body surface for a cut or abrasion from which blood may be transferred to a handkerchief.

Anaesthetic areas

The patient is blindfolded and the areas mapped out. On retesting, the areas will differ considerably.

Artificial oedema

Evidence of constriction of a limb may be present.

Artificial temperature

Take the temperature under actual observation and, if necessary, with another thermometer.

Deafness

A provocative remark made in an ordinary tone, such as the ordering of a strong purgative, or the addition or removal of some article of diet, may demonstrate that the patient has heard. The matter can always be cleared up by an aural surgeon or audiometrician using special tests (p. 136).

Dizziness

The Romberg test is performed (p. 132). In a genuine case the patient rocks or actually falls. If malingering is suspected, the attention of the patient is distracted, e.g. by asking him if he feels pin-pricks. In a genuine case the unsteadiness still persists, while in a fraudulent case it usually ceases.

If allowed to fall (the examiner having taken precautions to see that no injury can occur) the patient will slide to the ground rather than fall.

Loss of sight

Special tests by an ophthalmic surgeon readily expose a case of malingering of this type.

Mental symptoms

The symptoms do not conform to any of the recognised

mental disorders. The symptoms are only present when an observer is at hand.

Pain

An assumed pain differs in description on repeated questioning. If asked to indicate the painful spot it will be found that this area can be pressed on without complaint of pain later in the examination. Movements alleged to be impracticable on account of pain are performed painlessly in another way—thus if he says he cannot stoop down, he can probably sit up in bed and lean well forward—an action which produces the same degree of movement.

Paralysis of a limb

The patient may resist passive movements. If the limb is held up there is a momentary pause before it drops. The reflexes are normal and there is no wasting.

Skin conditions

Artificial lesions produced by fingernails, forks, pumice stone, etc, are found in areas easily accessible to the right hand, are longitudinal in form, and not usually found on the face, hands or genital organs.

If any suspected case of malingering is indefinite, a strict regime of low diet, no smoking or reading will usually soon indicate whether the symptoms are genuine or not.

DRUNKENNESS

Evidence may be gained from the patient's appearance and behaviour. There may be abnormalities in the clothing, speech and gait. Injection of the conjunctiva and tremors may be present. Questions may be asked as to date, place and time, and an account of various happenings. Tests may be given in respect of coordinating and writing. The smell of alcohol in the breath is not very reliable in itself. Conditions somewhat resembling drunkenness may be produced by some drugs and substances such as insulin. With the patient's permission blood and urine may be collected and sent to the laboratory for alcohol estimation (pp. 80 and

170). Using a breathalyser the subject's breath can be analysed for its alcohol content.

POISONING

In a case of suspected poisoning it is first necessary to exclude corrosive poisoning. The lips, upper surface of tongue and pharynx are examined for the marks of strong corrosives. If there is no evidence of corrosive poisoning a stomach tube should be passed and the stomach emptied. The stomach is then washed out with successive small quantities of water (about 250 to 300ml). It should be repeated at least six times or until the washings are clear. The stomach contents and washings are kept for subsequent examination. Any vomit, urine or faeces should be kept in case required. It is also important to find, if possible, the glass or bottle from which the poison has been taken.

Investigation for bacterial food poisoning is described on p. 38. In suspected drug overdose a 10ml sample of clotted blood should be sent to the laboratory (p. 87).

LEAD POISONING

Minute quantities of lead are excreted by normal individuals. In cases of suspected lead poisoning the following examinations may be carried out:

1. *Haemoglobin and blood film.* Lead poisoning produces anaemia and stippling of the red cells.

2. *Urine for lead and coproporphyrin.* A complete 24-hour urine is collected. Lead excretion of over 1mg per day suggests lead poisoning. There is also increased coproporphyrin excretion.

3. *Blood lead level.* This should be less than 2μmol/litre (40μg/100ml). Blood lead assay detects subclinical poisoning. Clinical effects only become evident with levels of $3-4\mu$mol/litre ($60-80\mu$g/100ml). Levels of $5-8\mu$mol/litre ($100-160\mu$g/100ml) are seen in lead encephalopathy and can be fatal.

Vitamin Deficiencies

VITAMIN A

Normally, blood contains $0.7-7\mu$mol/litre ($20-200\mu$g/100ml). This can be estimated chemically, 10ml of heparinised or clotted blood being required. Deficiency can also be detected by the *dark adaptation test* which shows impairment when the blood level falls below 0.35μmol/litre (10μg/100ml). Deficiency occurs in intestinal malabsorption, excessive use of liquid paraffin and dietary deficiency.

VITAMIN B_1

Normally blood pyruvic acid is $0.045-0.110$mmol/litre ($0.4-1.0$mg/100ml). In deficiency of vitamin B_1 the figure is raised. (See Blood Pyruvic Acid and Pyruvic Tolerance Test, p. 99.)

VITAMIN B_{12}

Normally blood serum contains $0.11-0.44$nmol/litre ($150-600$pg/ml) of vitamin B_{12}. In pernicious anaemia and subacute combined degeneration of the cord this figure is greatly reduced. It is also reduced in the intestinal malabsorption syndromes (together with folic acid, iron and vitamin D), in some cases of carcinoma of stomach and occasionally in megaloblastic anaemia of pregnancy. Often vitamin B_{12} deficiency can be inferred, as in typical pernicious anaemia by the megaloblastic bone marrow, histamine-fast achlorhydria and slightly raised serum bilirubin. Confirmation should be obtained by microbiological assay before starting therapy. The laboratory should be informed of any recent antibiotic (including antituberculous) or cytotoxic therapy, which can give false low results.

Microbiological assay

5–10ml of clotted blood is collected, preferably using a new syringe, needle and universal container. (Minute traces of contamination can vitiate the assay.) The vitamin B_{12} is estimated in the laboratory by measuring the amount of growth of a specially chosen micro-organism produced by different dilutions of the patient's serum.

Other tests for vitamin B_{12} deficiency

1. *Therapeutic Response.* Administration of vitamin B_{12} to a patient with pernicious anaemia produces a reticulocytosis (see p. 49) on about the fifth day, detected by serial reticulocyte counts. This is followed by a steady rise in the haemoglobin level.

2. *Schilling* or *Dicopac Test* (p. 18). Using radioactive B_{12} it is possible to diagnose pernicious anaemia even in a patient who has been receiving treatment.

FOLIC ACID

Blood folic acid can be estimated by microbiological assay, collection of the specimen being as for vitamin B_{12}. Normally the blood level, reported as serum folate, is more than 5.7μmol/litre (2.5μg/ml). Certain drugs cause a false low result and the laboratory must be informed of any recent antibiotic or cytotoxic therapy. In deficiency, e.g. megaloblastic anaemia of pregnancy and the malabsorption syndrome, it disappears from the blood more rapidly than normal after intravenous administration. This is the basis of the folic acid clearance test. Absorption after oral administration may similarly be tested. In folic acid deficiency, the bone marrow characteristically contains 'intermediate megaloblasts'. This is a useful aid to diagnosis. (See FIGLU, p. 173.)

VITAMIN C (Ascorbic Acid)

Deficiency is present in scurvy and in some cases of gastric ulcer which have had prolonged medical treatment. Deficiency can be detected by the ascorbic acid saturation test. After at least 3 hours fasting the patient drinks an ascorbic acid solution. This contains 11mg of ascorbic acid per kilogram body-weight, i.e. a total of about 700mg of ascorbic acid for an adult, dissolved in about 150ml of water. The bladder is emptied at exactly 4 hours after the drink and the urine discarded. The bladder is again emptied exactly 2 hours later and the 2-hour specimen of urine sent to the laboratory. Normally about 0.8mg/kg is excreted, i.e. about 50mg in adults. In vitamin C deficiency a total of about 3mg or less is excreted. When excretion is found to be deficient the test is repeated on several consecutive days. Even normal people may not be fully saturated with vitamin C initially. For blood ascorbic acid, see p. 82.

VITAMIN D

The normal serum level of 25 hydroxycholecalciferol is 3.5–30µg/litre in adults and children. In rickets and osteomalacia the level may be too low to be detectable. In intoxication from over-dosage of vitamin D, serum levels exceed 400µg/litre. For its estimation 10ml of clotted blood are required.

VITAMIN K

The prothrombin time is raised, i.e. the prothrombin ratio increased, in vitamin K deficiency, e.g. obstructive jaundice and haemorrhagic disease of the newborn. The prothrombin ratio (p. 54) is also increased in patients treated by anticoagulants such as warfarin, phenindione (Dindevan), nicoumalone (Sinthrome) and ethylbiscoumacetate (Tromexan). The effect of these drugs is counteracted by vitamin K.

Speech Tests

Disturbances of speech can be divided into those affecting language, voice and articulation.

TESTS FOR LANGUAGE DISTURBANCE (e.g. Dysphasia and Aphasia)

These are tests used by speech therapists to assess what kind of language dysfunction exists, e.g. whether of comprehension (receptive) or of expression (expressive or executive) or both (global or mixed). Ability to read, write and calculate is also tested. There are also language attainment tests for children, e.g. Peabody and English vocabulary scales.

VOICE ASSESSMENT

At the present time this is generally assessed by auditory perception, which is necessarily subjective. If an abnormality is suspected the patient is referred to an ENT specialist, e.g. for rhinoscopy (p. 117), auriscopy (p. 137), and laryngoscopy (p. 119).

TESTS FOR THE DISTURBANCE OF ARTICULATION

Defects of articulation take the form of distortions, substitutions, omissions and transpositions of sounds. They may be caused by:

(a) Neuromuscular disturbance (dysarthria), detected by neurological examination.

(b) Structural defect such as cleft palate, detected by examination of the oral cavity.

(c) Mental deficiency, detected by developmental screening tests (p. 139).

(d) Emotional disturbance, usually detected by case history.

(e) Imitation of speech, also usually detected by case history.

(f) Hearing loss, detected by screening tests, e.g. by testing reaction to noise, and in some cases by audiometric tests (p. 136). In order to assess articulation in children an Articulation Attainment Test (e.g. Renfrew) may be used.

Index